Childhood Tuberculosis:
Modern Imaging and Clinical Concepts

Springer
Berlin
Heidelberg
New York
Barcelona
Budapest
Hong Kong
London
Milan
Paris
Tokyo

Bryan J. Cremin and Douglas H. Jamieson

Childhood Tuberculosis: Modern Imaging and Clinical Concepts

With 141 Figures

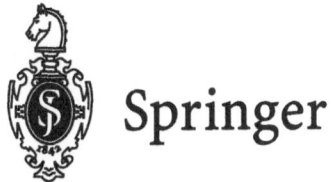 Springer

Bryan J. Cremin, MD (Cape Town), FRCR, FRACR
University of Cape Town, Department of Paediatric Radiology,
Red Cross Children's Hospital, Cape Town 7700, South Africa

Douglas H. Jamieson, M. Med, FF(Rad D)SA
Red Cross Children's Hospital, Cape Town 7700, South Africa

Cover illustrations: Ch. 3, Fig. 14b: IV contrast-enhanced CT. Ch. 4, Fig. 21d: Coronal IV gadolinium-enhanced MR. Ch. 5, Fig. 2c: Ultrasound – nodes at celiac axis. Ch. 6, Fig. 13a: Sagittal T2 MR showing complete destruction of the bodies of T10-T11.

ISBN-13: 978-1-4471-3013-0   e-ISBN-13: 978-1-4471-3011-6
DOI: 10.1007/978-1-4471-3011-6
British Library Cataloguing in Publication Data
Cremin, Bryan J.
  Childhood Tuberculosis: Modern Imaging
  and Clinical Concepts
  I. Title II. Jamieson, Douglas H.
  618.92995

Library of Congress Cataloging-in-Publication Data
Cremin, B.J. (Bryan Joseph), 1929–
    Childhood tuberculosis: modern imaging and clinical concepts /
Bryan J. Cremin and Douglas H. Jamieson.
        p. cm.
  Includes bibliographical references and index.
                    (alk. paper)
  1. Tuberculosis in children. I. Jamieson, Douglas H. II. Title.
  [DNLM: 1. Tuberculosis – in infancy & childhood. 2. Diagnostic
Imaging – in infancy & childhood. WF 415 C915c 1995]
RC312.6.C4C74 1995
618.92′995—dc20
DNLM/DLC   95–7046
for Library of Congress   CIP

Typeset by EXPO Holdings, Malaysia

28/3830-543210   Printed on acid-free paper

Dedication

To our most important heritage, the children of this world, their continued good health and salvation from infectious diseases. In this we include our own daughters Geraldine, Gabriella and Cristina and grandchildren Lara and Ryan.

BJC and DHJ

Dedication

Foreword

In 1967 Dr Bryan Cremin arrived in South Africa to head the Department of Diagnostic Radiology at the Red Cross Children's Hospital, and became the first specialist paediatric radiologist on the faculty of the University of Cape Town. Now, in 1994, Professor Cremin is internationally recognised, and, just before his retirement, has, with the support of his colleagues, summarised his 27 years of experience of tuberculosis in southern Africa.

Tuberculosis is an extraordinary infection – ancient, gaining a sinister reputation and at times occurring in disastrous epidemics. By affecting both princes and poets, children and the aged, it has altered the course of history. But, the effects aside, the methods which have been used to treat tuberculosis over the centuries are as remarkable as any in the folklore of medicine. Even in the relatively short period in which radiography has been available, treatment has been, by today's standards, somewhat unusual. For example, it was deemed important to "rest" the diseased lung and to collapse any tuberculous cavity. Lacking CT-, MRI- or ultra-sound techniques, radiologists were nevertheless expert at recognising wax or dental compound which had been blindly injected into a cavity, and in distinguishing ping-pong balls in the pleural space from a pneumothorax with adhesions. If air in the pleura did not collapse the lung (or even both lungs in some patients), then air or gas was used to produce a pneumoperitoneum; to help, the hemidiaphragm was often paralysed temporarily or permanently, depending on the skill of the operator who crushed the phrenic nerve. If all else failed, ribs were shortened and the chest wall was collapsed surgically. All this usually took place in a breezy or chilly sanatorium, often at high altitude. Many patients recovered, but a large number did not, and recurrences or relapses were frequent. In children, the diagnosis of tuberculosis was often a death sentence. Why was it that beautiful, fair-haired 3-year-olds seemed to be so susceptible to tuberculous meningitis? Once diagnosed, parents and physicians knew that they could but watch hopelessly for the 3–6 weeks of life that remained. There was no cure.

Tuberculosis was so nearly conquered when streptomycin and other drugs became available in the 1940s, but the infection persisted and has again become a major cause of ill-health and death, fuelled by malnutrition, migration, addictions and AIDS. In Europe and North America it used to be regarded as a "chronic" disease, but anyone who has worked in Africa (or other similar regions) will have realised that tuberculosis is often an acute, even fulminating, infection which may rapidly affect the lungs, skeleton or any other part of the body. Now AIDS and other causes of immunosuppression have brought this aspect of tuberculosis to all communities.

Professor Cremin and his colleagues have re-emphasised the protean pattern, or indeed the lack of consistent patterns, which is one of the characteristics of tuberculosis. They have described and illustrated superbly what may be expected, both clinically and on imaging. Nevertheless, they will be the first to admit that tuberculosis will continue to surprise even the most experienced, suddenly appearing in ways that are quite out-of-character. This is the message this book so clearly conveys. There are distinct and recognisable profiles of pulmonary or other tuberculous infections, but there are also many other presentations which so closely resemble some other infections, or even tumours, and which are so unlike tuberculosis that the imaging and clinical diagnosis is in doubt and the laboratory reports are viewed with disbelief.

The message is simple: do not forget tuberculosis whenever there is something odd in the way an illness progresses. In such cases, as this book illustrates so well, conventional imaging may not be enough, and newer methods may solve a diagnostic impasse. In these days of drug resistance and atypical myobacteria, time wasted in establishing the correct diagnosis may prove fatal, not only to the patient but also to relatives and contacts. The chronic illness which could be contemplated for a year or two, because time was part of the healing art, is no longer so co-operative.

Professor Cremin and his colleagues have produced an eminently readable and fully illustrated book which will be of immediate assistance to all who must recognise and treat this infinitely changeable infection. Whatever other changes may occur in the saga of tuberculosis, the principles laid down will still guide the choice of the appropriate diagnostic imaging. With the right techniques, much more can be learned quickly and the choice and timing of treatment, including surgery where necessary, can be better judged. But above all else, this book will increase our awareness of the manifold varieties of this ancient affliction, which has once more become of such major importance, especially, but not only, in Africa. It is no exaggeration to say that tuberculosis is once again changing the course of history in many countries. This record of many years of experience has been written at a most appropriate time.

P.E.S. Palmer, MD, FRCP, FRCR
Emeritus Professor of Radiology
The University of California
Davis, USA
Previously Professor of Radiology
The University of Cape Town, South Africa

Preface

I have always been interested in tuberculosis; my father had sanatorium treatment and three members of my class at Medical School contracted the disease. In those days there was some social stigma attached to the disease, and patients had to be isolated from "normal" folk. Although at that time effective drugs had already been discovered, they were not freely obtainable in the post-World-War-II period; famous authors, such as George Orwell (the originator of the sinister "Big Brother"), had to invoke the help of the British Minister of Health to get supplies of streptomycin from the USA. Subsequently a variety of powerful drugs became more freely available and were used in effective combination to treat tuberculosis. With them the belief grew that the disease would no longer present a problem in Western countries. Some of the fallacies of this prediction are mentioned in our introductory chapter to this volume. On the Continent of Africa the disease has always remained a problem and for the 27 years that I have practiced radiology in South Africa, tuberculosis has remained our largest infectious disease problem. The disease has also persisted and expanded in Asia, and we have tried to reflect this situation in our reference survey. Unfortunately, however, some of the literature from countries such as India has not been freely available to us in our libraries.

Another reason for writing is that it has been some years since a book on childhood TB has been written. The two seminal books both entitled *Tuberculosis in Children* were written in 1963 by Lincoln and Sewel[1] and by Miller, Seal and Taylor[2], and Miller added a further edition to the series *Medicine in the Tropics* in 1982[3]. Since then radiology and imaging have made huge advances and it is within this framework that this book was gestated with the hope that physicians and radiologists would be helped by descriptions, current imaging technology and illustrations of diagnostic findings. The efficacy of treatment is dependant on early diagnosis, but a misdiagnosis, besides being a human tragedy, can result in serious legal complications. It is hoped that our experience may be of help to physicians in other countries who have less experience of tuberculosis among their patients.

There are many aspects of this age-old disease that are still not understood, particularly in its pathogenesis and human protective mechanisms. Radiologically, I am sometimes puzzled by the fact that there is usually a single pulmonary focus although multiple bacteria must have been inhaled. We have followed the established concept that although the initial lesion is parenchymal, its progression and complications in the lung are mainly lymphobronchial. The words "glands" (from the Latin *glans*, an acorn) and "nodes" (*nodus*, knot) are interchangeable, and as the word "tubercle" derives from the Latin *tuber* (knots or nodules), we have given preference to the term nodes to describe adenopathy. The differentiation between hematogenous and bronchogenic spread is sometimes difficult to establish radiologically and both forms of dissemination may exist at the same time. Moreover, the disease, besides being a morbus miseriae, may be morbus per corpus, wide-spread at an early stage and flaring up in extrapulmonary sites, sometimes well after the initial pulmonary infection has apparently subsided. The relationship between the primary infection and so-called post-primary infection are complex questions that remain largely unanswered and remain as clinical concepts.

I am most grateful to my clinical colleague Professor M. Ehlers for throwing some light on the behaviour and microbiology of *M. tuberculosis* and to both Professors M. Kibel and P. Donald for their contributions and experienced insight into modern diagnosis and treatment. I am also most grateful for the support of all of my clinical colleagues at the Red Cross Children's Hospital, and particularly to the members of my department. I am especially indebted to my co-author Dr D.H. Jamieson for his unbounded enthusiasm in collecting and collating much of the modern imaging material which I hope will be the feature of this book. He has kept me up to date with some of the recent technical advances and without his assistance this book would never have been completed. To Mrs Joyce Green goes my gratitude for her perpetual patience in typing and retyping our often illegible writing.

Finally I would like to acknowledge Dr H. Goodman (Figs 3.30, 3.31) and Dr C. Stoyanov (Fig. 6.9b) for providing illustrations in adolescents. All the other illustrations are from our hospital and concern children under the age of 13 years. We would like to acknowledge the use of illustrations from our own publications, in *Pediatric Radiology* (Figs 3.7, 3.33, 3.36 and 3.37), *British Journal of Radiology* (Figs 5.15, 5.20, 6.21, 6.27 and 6.29) and *British Journal of Bone and Joint Surgery* (Figs 6.5, 6.7 and 6.8).

References

1. Lincoln EM, Sewel EM (1963) Tuberculosis in Children. New York: McGraw-Hill
2. Miller FJW, Seal RME, Taylor MD (1963) Tuberculosis in Children. Edinburgh: Churchill
3. Miller FJW (1982) Tuberculosis in Children. Evolution, Epidemiology, Treatment and Prevention. Medicine in the Tropics. Edinburgh: Churchill Livingstone.

Cape Town   B.J. Cremin
October 1994

Contents

Contributors

Professor Mario R.W. Ehlers, MBChB, PhD
Department of Medical Biochemistry
University of Cape Town Medical School
7925 Observatory
South Africa

Professor Maurice A. Kibel, FRCP, DCH
ICH Building
Red Cross Children's Hospital
7700 Rondebosch
South Africa

Professor Peter R. Donald, MD, FCP, MRCP, DCH, DTM&H
Department of Paediatrics and Child Health
Faculty of Medicine
PO Box 19063
7505 Tygerberg
South Africa

1 Historical and Pathological Background of Tuberculosis

B.J. Cremin

Historical and Epidemiological Aspects

The "white plague", as Oliver Wendell Holmes (1861) named tuberculosis, has infected man for as long as historical records exist. Lesions have been found in the vertebrae of neolithic man (5000 BC) and in Egyptian mummies (3700 BC). Recent DNA studies on a Peruvian mummy have shown conclusive evidence that pulmonary tuberculosis existed in the Americas centuries before the arrival of Columbus[1]. Tuberculosis remains man's greatest killer from infectious diseases and currently affects more than 20% of the world's population. Every year there are 8–10 million new cases and 3–5 million deaths attributed to tuberculosis[2]. The World Health Organization is concerned about the situation[3], especially in children. There are 1.3 million infected children under the age of 15 years and 450,000 die annually[4,5]. These children, infected by adults, represent a reservoir from which future generations will be afflicted[5].

Classical non-medical literature includes graphic accounts of the disease. John Bunyan (1680) described the life and death of Mr Badman as, "The Captain of all these men of death that came to take him away, was the consumption, for it was that which brought him down to the grave", and the coughing that Hans Castorp heard in *The Magic Mountain* was described in the Nobel Prize winning novel by Thomas Mann (1924) as "It was coughing, obviously a man coughing like no other he had ever heard, and compared with which any other had been a magnificent and healthy manipulation of life; a coughing that had no conviction and gave no relief, that did not even come out in paroxysms, but was just a feeble dreadful welling up of juices of organic dissolution".

Although the disease, throughout the ages, has flourished in over-crowded environments, it has afflicted not only the poor but also government leaders, distinguished physicians, scientists, artists and writers, too numerous to mention individually.

Historically the word pthisis appears early in Greek medical writings, but this was a non-specific term to describe wasting away. Consumption, a Latin word, became the popular term for tuberculosis in the seventeenth century. Similar descriptive terms have been used world-wide with the biblical Hebrew "Schachepeth", the Urdu, "Tabay diq", the Pathan, "Nare maraz" and the Hindu "Xoy" or waning of the moon. Richard Morton (1637–1698) who died of the disease, noted the different forms of pulmonary consumption in his prestigious volumes *Phthisiologia*. He did not understand the true nature of the disease but his descriptive accounts are graphic.

A Consumptive Cough is a dry cough proceeding from a *Glandulous Swelling or Tubercle of the Lungs themselves ... On the contrary, a Simple Catarrh cough owes its Origin from a distillation of rheum* cut out, as it were, in continual drops by the Uvula and Almonds and the other Glands seated in the upper part of the Wind-pipe, yea, and by all the Glandulous Coat of the Wind-pipe itself.

Interesting comments on the fundamental principles of infectious disease control were well articulated in 1513, not by a physician, but by the political scientist Nicolla Machievelli[6].

It happens then as it does to physicians in the treatment of Consumption, which in the commencement is easy to cure and difficult to understand; but when it has neither been discovered in due time nor treated upon a proper principle, it becomes easy to understand and difficult to cure. The same thing happens in state affairs; by foreseeing them at a distance, which is only done by men of talents, the evils which might arise from them are soon cured; but when, from want of foresight, they are suffered to increase to such a height that they are perceptible to everyone, there is no longer any remedy.

Franciscus Sylvius (1614–1672) conceived the term tuberculosis when he described the characteristic lung nodules as "tubercules" (L. *tuber*, knots or nodules) and observed their eventual evolution into lung cavities. However, many pathologists, including Rudolph Virchov, the great protagonist of cellular disease, initially believed the condition to be constitutional, involving a form of tumor, spreading to the lungs and causing calcareous ulcers.

Theophilus Bonetus (1628–1689) of Geneva collected a large amount of pathological material (3000 cases) in his book *Serpulchretum Sive Anatomica Practica*. Amongst these are 150 cases in which the described pathology is typical of tuberculosis. A French physician, Jean Jacques Manget, reproduced this book in 1700 and added a personal description of the minute granulations (grandines) disseminated throughout the body; he was the first to compare them to millet seeds (Magnitudine Seminum Milli) thus introducing the term miliary tuberculosis.

The first recorded speculation that tuberculosis might be communicable was by Benjamin Martin (1772) who suggested the germs or what he calls a "amaliculae or their seed which are inimicable to our nature" were transmitted by a breath emitted from the lung. However, the first proof that tuberculosis was an infective disease was by the French physician, Jean Antoin Villemin (1827–1892). He was professor in the Institute of Military Hygiene at Val-de-Grace and noted that young soldiers from the country were more likely to develop pulmonary tuberculosis after being confined to crowded barracks. He induced tuberculosis in rabbits by inoculating them with human pus and infected fluids. This monumental finding was ignored until the great German scientist Robert Koch, in 1882, astonished the world, not only by histologically staining *Mycobacterium tuberculosis*, but culturing it from crushed tubercules.

Although a primary inoculation of guinea pigs with tubercle bacilli in the skin produced a non-healing ulcer, Koch noted that reinoculation of the animals after several weeks produced only a firm, red nodule that eventually healed (the Koch phenomenon). This first suggested an existence of immunity to infection. Unfortunately, in 1890 he also announced that culture filtrates cured the disease, a claim that was promptly discredited. Koch refused to divulge the nature and preparation of the "curative" material – an action imputed by some to the wish to assure a monopoly for the German government and to acquire an institute for himself. Nevertheless, those infiltrates, later partially purified, became used for tuberculin skin testing, which remains a principal means to establish that infection has occurred.

The landmark description of the pulmonary focus and its regional gland involvement was by the Viennese pathologist Anton Ghon (1912). He also emphasized, as did the New York pathologist Edith Lincoln (1935), that rapid hematogenous spread was a feature of tuberculosis in children.

During the eighteenth and early nineteenth centuries between 20% and 30% of the deaths in urban districts of Europe and America were due to tuberculosis and it became established that the disease proliferated when over-crowding and poor socio-economic conditions prevailed. The disease progressed into urban areas following mass industrial migrations for work both in Europe and America. Before World War I the disease was the major cause of death in children in Vienna with 33% of 3200 autopsies having active tuberculosis. In the peace-time Warsaw of 1938 the disease was less common in Jews (who were at the time considered to have some racial immunity) than in Gentiles. This changed with gross over-crowding in the ghettos and the figures reversed with a rise from 71/100,000 in 1938 to 205/100,000 in 1940 and 601/100,000 in 1942[7].

In America, Dr Ernest Livingstone Trudeau, himself a sufferer from tuberculosis, established the importance of the environment in modifying reaction to the disease. He inoculated rabbits with the bacillus and found that those exposed to sunlight and nutritious food had a better rate of survival. He set up the first American sanatorium next to the beautiful Saranac Lake in the Adirondacks, north of New York. Many sanatoria became famous and amongst these was the "Magic Mountain" at Davos in Switzerland. The main treatment was a balanced diet, fresh air and bed rest. Although some recovered, for many it was only a long and lingering horizontal death sentence.

In 1943 in the USA Albert Schatz and Selman Waksman showed that the bacterial antibiotic streptomycin, derived from the soil actinomycete streptomyces griseus, was effective against *M. tuberculosis*. In Sweden during the following year, Jorgen Lehmann showed that para-aminosalicilic acid (PAS), which is related to the humble aspirin, could be used with advantage in association with streptomycin. There have been many workers in anti-tuberculosis drug research and with the discovery of even more powerful drugs and the benefit of combined therapies the eventual eradication of tuberculosis was predicted[8]. A sense of euphoria ensued and in 1971 at a symposium held in London, it was considered that although it was unwise to be complacent about the future incidence of tuberculosis it was also unwise not to be realistic. The conclusion was that not only would tuberculosis be rare in the UK by 1990 but that by the year 2010 it would only be of interest to the medical historian[8]. This prediction was incorrect, as an alarming resurgence of tuberculosis in large urban areas both in the UK[9] and in the USA has occurred and the disease has again become a major health concern[10,11,12,13,14]. This increase has mainly been reported in intravenous drug users, HIV-positive persons, prison in-mates and the elderly in nursing homes[12]. Factors considered responsible are the discontinuation of anti-tuberculosis health measures, and over-crowded living conditions for immigrants and refugees from countries where tuberculosis is endemic[15]. Other reasons include poor physician/patient compliance[16], making drug regimes less effective, and the increasing prevalence of drug-resistant organisms, particularly to the two most effective drugs isoniazid and rifampicin[17]. The stark reality world-wide was that by 1990 it was estimated that there were 8 million new cases a year with 3 million deaths. Approximately one-third of the world's population is infected with *M. tuberculosis* and therefore at risk for developing the disease[6]. The majority of these cases are in Africa and Asia so that tuberculosis remains man's greatest infectious disease killer, causing 6.7% of all deaths in the developing world, and 18.5% of the deaths all adults aged between 15 and 59 years[6].

There has also been a World-wide increase in tuberculosis in children. Figures for 1990 from the USA showed an increase, in children less than 15 years, of 30% in 1987 and 29% in 1989, and 59% occurred in the group traditionally at the highest risk, that is infants and children less than 5 years of age[5]. In the USA about 80% of pediatric tuberculosis occurs in minority groups and there has been a marked increase in over-crowded urban areas[18,19,20]. Although the majority of these children were born in the USA, the proportion of foreign-born children is increasing. In Cape Town, South Africa, the incidence has risen to 679 per 100,000 and the condition remains the most common infectious disease[21].

Factors other than poor nutrition and socio-economic factors depress immunity to tuberculosis and the current concern is in HIV-immunocompromized hosts. This is a world-wide problem[19], but particularly in Central Africa[22]. In South Africa and the UK AIDS has yet to make its full impact on children, but it would be folly to think it will not come.

The combination of HIV and tuberculosis is associated with an increased incidence of extrapulmonary infections[23,24]. AIDS also precipitates an increased incidence of other mycobacterial and fungus diseases[25] which further increases the burden of tuberculosis.

Further Historical Reading

Brown L (1941) The story of clinical pulmonary tuberculosis. Baltimore: Williams and Wilkins

Castiglioni A (1941) A history of medicine. New York: Aknopf

Coonavia HM, Benetar SR (1991) A century of tuberculosis: South African perspectives. Cape Town: Oxford University Press

Cummins SL (1949) Tuberculosis in history from the seventeenth century to our own times. London: Baillière, Tindall and Co

Dubos R, Dubos J (1953) The white plague. Boston: Little, Brown and Co

Mann T (1928) The magic mountain, English Edn. London: Martin Secker and Warburg Ltd

Packard RM (1989) White plague, black labor: tuberculosis and the political economy of health and disease in South Africa. Berkeley University: of California Press

Ryan F (1992) Tuberculosis: the greatest story never told. Bromsgrove, Worcestershire, England: Swift Publishers

Basic Pathology and Further Considerations

Tuberculous infection in humans occurs predominantly by inhalation of air-borne bacilli of 3–5 μm, which lodge in the pulmonary acinus to set up a chain of reactions. The mycobacteria require a high oxygen concentration for their growth but they may settle anywhere in the lungs in single or multiple foci. In children, depending on the immune reaction of the child, the disease may be localized and confined to lung parenchyma and adjacent lymph nodes, or become rapidly disseminated to other parts of the body. This is primary tuberculosis, i.e., the first infection which may pass clinically unrecognised in well-nourished, previously healthy children. When the disease is not contained at its initial focus or satellite lesions proliferate, the condition becomes progressive primary tuberculosis. Reactivation of disease or, less commonly, reinfection, in an immune-competent host will cause secondary or "adult" tuberculosis. Primary and secondary disease belong to the same spectrum and clear separation is not always possible, but the primary type is associated with enlargement of lymph nodes in the chest. This is not so in the "adult" type which is also more prone to fibrosis and cavitation and has a predelection for the upper lung zones.

The pathological pattern of development that follows has been well documented[26,27,28] and the following general stages, with which the time relations are not clear-cut, have been worked out in animal experiments.

I   An immediate host reaction with a localized collection of fluid and alveolar polymorphonuclear leukocytes which phagocytize but do not kill the bacillus.

II   A rapid, within 24-h, replacement of leukocytes by macrophages, histiocytes and macrophage-derived cells that form the Langerhans multinucleated giant cells. These form a focus of consolidation in which the phagocytized bacilli continue to multiply.

III   Within the next week or two the macrophages become elongated and partially fused to form the typical epithelioid cell tubercle or giant cell macrophage with an accumulation of peripheral lymphocytes.

IV   Necrosis of the central portion of this lesion occurs at about the end of the second week. The necrosis may fail to liquefy and persists as a caseous material, forming caseating granulomas. The lymphocytes are activated at this stage to attack the tubercle bacilli and release lymphocytes that attract more macrophages in an attempt to destroy the bacilli. It is at the stage of necrosis that a variety of antibodies develop in the serum and the cutaneous tuberculin test becomes positive.

V   The healing stages may occur after about a month. This is when fibrocytes appear at the periphery of the lesion and lay down dense interlacing strands of collagenous tissue that envelop the lesion. Within this capsule the tubercle bacillus may die or lie viable and dormant for long periods.

Coincident with these changes two separate immunological changes occur. Firstly, the infected person becomes tuberculous-positive, that is, hypersensitive to tuberculoprotein. Secondly, a varying degree of cellular immunity develops which is responsible for the inhibition and possible destruction of virulent tubercle bacilli. If there is a breakdown of cellular immunity, growth of tubercle bacilli occurs to the point where enough tuberculoprotein is produced to elicit a local necrotizing allergic reaction. Primary tuberculosis is a condition that reflects an individual's conversion from insensitivity to the tubercle bacillus proteins to positive reaction to them, and as such it is a disease of altered sensitivity or allergy[29]. The inflammatory response and necrosis are the result of a host cell-mediated immune response to the lung bacilli rather than the result of toxins of tissue-destroying enzymes by the bacteria[30].

At an early stage, before necrosis and fibrotic healing has occurred, the bacillus may, under certain conditions, spread through the body by hematogeneous, lymphatic or ingested sputum pathways. Certain organs and tissues are notably resistant to further multiplication of the bacilli at this stage; for example, the bone marrow, liver and spleen, though seeded with mycobacteria, are not usually sites of uncontrolled multiplication. Other sites, such as the brain, may have environments that favour the growth of bacilli, and numerous bacterial divisions may occur before specific immunity develops to limit replication[30]. The reaction is governed by the host's immune response and specific messenger proteins or cytokines such as tumor necrosis factor and interferon gamma tend to wall off the tubercles into localized granulomas. These granulomas are attempts by the body to restrict the spread of disease, but the necrosis also causes damage to the lung tissue so that there is a delicate balance between defense and destructive mechanisms. Local extension will occur by erosion through the initial enveloping capsule and results in further layers being laid down to form a larger tuberculous lesion. This extension is the basis of the formation of tuberculomas in which there are multiple concentric layers around a mass which is essentially caseous or cheesy. The nature of this necrosis may vary in different sites, e.g., a gumatous or more solid necrosis may occur in brain tuberculomas. Furthermore, tuberculomas may enlarge by themselves or react with adjacent tubercles to form large tuberculous masses which may become confluent.

There are two important aspects underlying tuberculosis pathogenesis, apart from the initial pulmonary infection[25]. Firstly, the primary infection is associated with an early dissemination to multiple sites creating an occult potential for extrapulmonary involvement. Secondly, cell-mediated immunity (CMI) is responsible not only for control of the primary focus, but also to maintain lesions in a dormant state. In optimum circumstances over 95% of children will have no clinical symptoms or diagnosis. There is only approximately an 8%–10% incidence of reactivation and this usually occurs in the first 5 years of life[31].

HIV-positive patients have already been briefly referred to and will be considered again in Chapters 2, 3 and 7. When CMI is impaired by HIV infection, protein-calorie malnutrition, intercurrent virus infection, leukemia, diabetes or a massive infection in early childhood, particularly in an over-crowded, poverty-stricken environment, progressive primary tuberculosis develops as a continuation of Stage IV in which a massive extension of local lesions or wide-spread diffuse disease occurs. Transbronchial dissemination may occur as a result of cavitation or necrotic lymph node erosion into adjacent bronchi. Associated with impaired CMI, multiple small foci may occur within the lungs and further predispose to rapid hematogeneous spread. Depending on the degree of interplay with host resistance, the pathology of tuberculosis is a continuous process in which imaging may show the morphology at differing stages and in different tissues throughout the body[32].

Children with established pulmonary tuberculosis are sick, but the bacteriological confirmation of the diagnosis may be difficult. The investigation of social contacts is very important as skin tests may be negative in the early stages or in immune-compromised children. Bacteriological confirmation even under optimal conditions may be less than 40%[33]. A difference both in clinical features and bacteriological confirmation has been noted between infants and older children. Infants less than 1 year old have a higher incidence of respiratory symptoms and may have a higher yield of *M. tuberculosis* from gastric aspirates[33] with a surprisingly high figure of 75% having been recently reported[34]. Radiology is often the first positive step in making the diagnosis and modern imaging techniques have increased this potential. In the central nervous system, computed tomography (CT) and magnetic resonance imaging (MR) have become essential for diagnosis and treatment. In the chest and skeletal system, good conventional radiology remains fundamental but is now complemented by both CT and MR. When MR is referred to, we have mainly used spin-echo sequences with the terms T1 and T2 to denote the weighting of the signals. In the abdomen, ultrasound has made a great contribution as a cost-effective method of evaluation. Based on experience over many years at the University of Cape Town's Red Cross War Memorial Children's Hospital, the impact of these modern modalities will be described and illustrated in this volume.

Although the material will be children it should be recognized that primary tuberculosis also occurs in adults, especially those suffering from a debilitating disease. Based on the evidence of conversion of the PPD (purified protein derivative; a tuberculin preparation) test associated with clinical, radiological and bacteriological evidence, a figure of 56% for primary tuberculosis (19 out of 34 cases) has been recorded in a series of patients over the age of 18 years[35].

References

1. British Medical Journal (1994) News report. 308:808
2. Stylbo K, Rouillon A (1981) Estimated global incidence of smear-positive pulmonary tuberculosis: unreliability of officially reported figures on tuberculosis. Bull Int Union Tuberc 56: 118–125
3. Kochi A (1991) The global tuberculosis situation and the new control strategy of the World Health Organization. Tubercle 72: 1–6
4. EPI Update Supplement (1989) Childhood tuberculosis and BCG vaccine. Geneva: World Health Organization
5. Starke JR, Jacobs RF, Jereb J (1992) Resurgence of tuberculosis in children. J Pediatr 120: 839–855
6. Bloom BR, Murray CJL (1992) Tuberculosis: commentary on a reemergent killer. Science 257: 1055–1064
7. Ober WB (1983) Anton Ghon and his complex. Pathol Annu 2: 79–85
8. Bignall JR (1971) Tuberculosis in England and Wales in the next 20 years. Postgrad Med 47: 759–762
9. Watson J (1993) Tuberculosis in Britain today. Br Med J 306: 221
10. Buckner CB, Leithiser RE, Walker CW, Allison JW (1991) The changing epidemiology of tuberculosis and other microbacterial infections in the Untied States: implications for the radiologist. AJR 156: 255–264
11. Snider Jr. DE, Rieder HL, Combs D, Bloch AB, Hayden CH, Smith MHD (1988) Tuberculosis in children. Pediatr Infect Dis J 7: 271–278
12. Davis SD, Yankelevitz DF, Williams T, Henschke CI (1993) Pulmonary tuberculosis in immunocompromised hosts: epidemiological, clinical and radiological assessment. Semin Roentgen. 28: 119–130
13. MacGregor RR (1993) Tuberculosis: from history to current Management. Semin Roentgenol 28: 101–108
14. Miller WT, Miller Jr. WT (1993) Tuberculosis in the normal host: radiological findings. Semin Roentgenol 28: 109–118
15. Centres for Disease Control: A strategic plan for the elimination of tuberculosis in the United States. (1989) MMWR 38: 269–272
16. Grange JM, Festenstein F (1993) The human dimension of tuberculosis control. Tuberc Lung Dis 74: 219–222
17. Snider Jr. DE, Roper WL (1992) The New Tuberculosis. N Engl J Med 326: 703–705
18. Nemir RC, Krasinski K (1988) Tuberculosis in children and adolescents in the 1980s. Pediatr Infect Dis 7: 375–379
19. Agrons GA, Markowitz RI, Kramer SS (1993) Pulmonary tuberculosis in Children. Semin Roentgenol 28: 158–172
20. Inselman LS, EL-Maraghy, Evans HE (1981) Apparent resurgence of tuberculosis in urban children. Pediatrics 68: 647–649
21. Kustner HGV (1991) Tuberculosis in the Cape Province. Epidemiological Comments 18: 30
22. De Cock KM, Soro B, Coulibaly IM et al. (1992) Tuberculosis and HIV Infection in Sub-Saharan Africa. JAMA 208: 1581–1587
23. Nunn P, Odhiambo J, Elliott A (1960) Tuberculosis and HIV Infection. Lancet 1044
24. Berenguer J, Moreno S, Laguna F et al. (1992) Tuberculous meningitis in patients affected with human immunodeficiency virus. N Engl J Med 326: 668–672
25. Davis SD, Yankelevitz DF, Williams T, Hanschke CI (1993) Pulmonary Tuberculosis in immunocompromised hosts: epidemiological, clinical and radiological assessment. Semin Roentgenol 28: 119–130
26. Medlar EM (1955) The behaviour of pulmonary tuberculous lesions: a pathological study (Part II). Am Rev Tuberc 71: 1–244
27. Pratt PC (1979) Pathology of Tuberculosis. Semin Roentgenol 14: 196–203
28. Hacque AK (1990) The pathology and pathophysiology of mycobacterial infections. J Thoracic Imaging 5: 8–16
29. Caffey J (1988) Primary Pulmonary Tuberculosis. In Silverman F (ed), Pediatric X-Ray Diagnosis (8th Ed) Chicago: Year Book Publishers, pp 1210–1227

30. Bass JB, Farer LS, Hopewell PC, Jacobs RF, Snider DE (1990) Diagnostic standards and classification of tuberculosis. Am Rev Respir Dis 142: 725–735

31. MacGregor RR (1993) Tuberculosis: from history to management. Semin Roentgen 28: 101–108

32. Palmer PES (1979) Pulmonary tuberculosis – usual and unusual radiographic presentations. Semin Roentgenol 14: 204–248

33. Starke JR, Taylor-Watts KT (1989) Tuberculosis in the pediatric population of Houston, Texas. Pediatrics 84: 28–35

34. Vallejo JG, Ong LT, Starke JR (1994) Clinical features, diagnosis and treatment of tuberculosis in infants. Pediatrics 94: 1–7

35. Woodring JH, Vandivere HM, Fried AM, Dillon ML, Williams TD, Melvin IG (1986) Update. The radiographic features of pulmonary tuberculosis. AJR 146: 497–506

2 Biology of *Mycobacterium tuberculosis* and the Host–Pathogen Relationship

M.R.W. Ehlers

Introduction

Mycobacterium tuberculosis is the single most successful pathogen in the world today, infecting one-third of the world's population, and producing 8–10 million new cases of active tuberculosis and 3 million deaths annually. Moreover, this success is not a recent phenomenon, as tuberculosis afflicted the ancients and in all likelihood has been an unwelcome companion during much of modern man's evolution. Indeed, in 1882 Robert Koch, pronouncing on its significance, declared that "all diseases, particularly the most dreaded infectious diseases such as bubonic plague, Asiatic cholera, etc., must rank far behind tuberculosis"[1].

To what may we ascribe the singular success of tuberculosis (TB)? This is a question that cannot be answered at present, even though the bacillus was discovered over 100 years ago and it is one of the most intensely studied of human pathogens. However, the picture that is now beginning to emerge – although, so far, consisting only of fleeting glimpses – is of a pathogen with exceedingly subtle and ingenious strategies to overcome the prodigious defenses of the host. The molecular details of the TB bacillus' *modus operandi* are being exposed one by one by the power of recombinant DNA technology, which has been brought to bear on this problem since the mid-1980s.

Prior to that date, TB research had been in a slump, driven by the misguided impression that the disease had been conquered. While the impression may have been justified in the West, where the disease was declining at a steady rate of 5%–6% per year since 1953[1], it ignored the fact that in the developing world the disease was raging on unabated, and in some areas, notably sub-Saharan Africa, was and is reaching epidemic proportions. Indeed, even in the West the heady optimism – expressed in 1989 in a strategic plan in the USA that forecast the virtual elimination of TB by the year 2010[2] – was blunted by the sobering realization that the progressive decline in TB incidence had stopped in 1985 and has since been rising steadily[1]. Thus, in addition to its relentless progress in the developing world, TB is also making a comeback in the prosperous West, fueled by immigration from high-prevalence countries, outbreaks amongst increasing numbers of homeless and indigents in congregative facilities, and, above all, the world-wide AIDS epidemic[1,3,4]. Compounding this resurgence is the looming spectre of drug resistance, which is particularly acutely felt in the USA where in some cities, such as New York, the incidence of multi-drug-resistant (MDR) TB is in the order of 20%[1]. This is a potentially catastrophic development, since under the best circumstances treatment of MDR TB is only 50%–60% successful, while in HIV-infected individuals mortality reaches 90%[1].

Under the confluence of these developments, TB is once again recognized to be a major threat to public health, and the lethargy that has characterized the West's involvement in controlling this disease in the past few decades has been replaced by a renewed and intense interest. Driven by heightened funding from the public and corporate sectors, a wave of biomedical scientists, particularly molecular biologists, has entered the fray, and the introduction of modern molecular and cell biological methods to attack previously intractable problems could not be timelier. What follows is a brief outline of recent advances and current thinking about the nature of the organism, its interaction with host cells, the immune response, the genetics of host susceptibility, and prospects for improved vaccines and drugs.

Characteristics of *Mycobacterium tuberculosis*

Mycobacterium tuberculosis (*M.tb.*) was noted by early investigators to possess two peculiar characteristics: acid-fast staining and slow growth. A great deal of significance was attached to these properties, but as was recently reviewed[5], a basic molecular explanation for them remains lacking and their relevance in pathogenesis is speculative.

Mycobacteria are generally considered to be Gram-positive, acid- and alcohol-fast rods which are aerobic and non-spore forming, and are classified with the actinomycetes[6]. The prodigiously thick and waxy cell wall of mycobacteria has long added to the mystique of these organisms, but recent advances in its structural analysis[7] have revealed that, although it is unusual in detail, it cannot as a whole be regarded as unique[5]. In its basic design the wall resembles those of Gram-positives, although distinctly unusual is an outer layer of mycolic acids – extremely long-chain, branched fatty acids – that are primarily responsible for the waxy character of the envelope. Of central importance in the pathogenic mechanisms of *M.tb.* – in terms of host cell invasion, intracellular persistence, and the elicited host immune response (see below) – are the envelope-associated and secreted proteins. Although by now a large number have been identified[8], many remain unknown and the functions of most are obscure. Further advances in our understanding of *M.tb.* virulence mechanisms and the immune response critically depend on our determining the structure and functions of exported proteins[9,10].

Mycobacteria are divided into two groups: fast-growers and slow-growers[6]. Most of the pathogens, including *M.tb.*, are slow-growers, but efforts to link this characteristic convincingly to virulence have failed. For instance, within the so-called *M. tuberculosis* complex, the fastest-growing strains are the most virulent[11], whereas the avirulent vaccine strain *M. bovis* BCG is slow-growing. One of the outstanding questions we face today is: What is the relationship between dormancy, virulence, and slow growth? It is generally accepted conventional wisdom that *M.tb.* can enter a profound state of dormancy (or latency), persist in this state in the human host for years or decades and then, under favourable circumstances, reactivate and cause disease[3,12]. However, the evidence for this is largely circumstantial and, except for a few isolated reports[13], putative dormant bacilli have not been directly observed *in vitro* or *in vivo*, nor, for that matter, can any molecular explanation be offered for this phenomenon. If, as many believe, deep dormancy is a real phenomenon, then it is likely to contribute to the chronicity and difficulty in treating TB, in that dormant organisms may persist even after chemotherapy, with later recrudescence of the disease. This could be a particularly difficult problem in the HIV-infected patient.

The *M. tuberculosis*–Macrophage Interaction

Central to the pathogenicity and virulence of *M.tb.* is its invasion, survival, and growth within its host cell, the macrophage. *M.tb.* is a *facultative* intracellular parasite, preferentially growing intracellularly but also capable of extracellular growth, both within the host and in culture medium in the laboratory. Indeed, it is interesting that an organism that can easily survive extracellularly chooses to invade the macrophage, a hostile phagocytic cell that is key to the host's immune system. Invasion involves a series of events consisting of three critical steps: adherence; internalization; and intracellular survival[14].

Adherence of *M.tb.* to Macrophages

It is often assumed that because macrophages are "professional" phagocytic cells they will spontaneously engulf all encountered particles without a requirement for specific adhesion. Whereas this may be true for many inert particles, it is practically never true for dedicated intracellular macrophage parasites, and *M.tb.* is no exception. *M.tb.* has been shown to home in on a few restricted macrophage receptors, particularly the type 3 complement receptor (CR3)[15] (Fig. 2.1). This is highly significant because CR3 is a commonly used macrophage receptor, serving as the means of attachment for, inter alia, *Histoplasma capsulatum*, *Legionella pneu-*

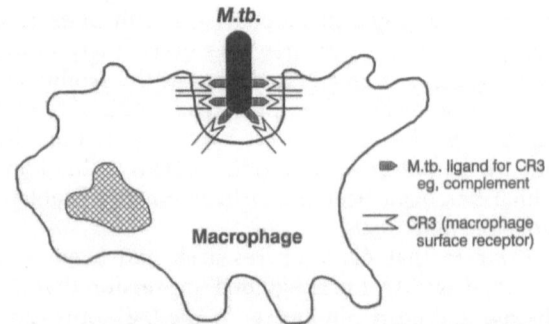

Fig. 2.1. Adherence to and invasion of macrophages by *M.tb.* Recent research indicates that *M.tb.* binds to specific receptors on the surface of macrophages, of which the most important is complement receptor type 3 (CR3). This involves the fixing of complement to the surface of the bacilli to provide a key (or ligand) that fits into the lock (CR3). It is likely that the use of CR3 for the invasion of macrophages provides *M.tb.* with a safe passage and prepares the ground for the subsequent occupation of a protected niche inside the cell (see Fig. 2.2).

mophila, Leishmania, and *Bordetella pertussis*[14]. CR3 belongs to a large family of surface proteins called *integrins* that are found on most mammalian cells and which are critical in promoting attachment (or *adhesion*) of cells to one another and to the extracellular matrix[16]. Thus, *M.tb.* and the other pathogens listed above exploit a system that is well established in mammalian cells for adhesion. Indeed, the subversion of host cell systems for the benefit of parasites is a common theme in the strategies used by intracellular pathogens[17].

M.tb. binds to the CR3 by (as would be expected) fixing complement (component C3) to its cell surface[15]. In addition it is possible that there are one or more specific surface proteins on *M.tb.* that can bind to CR3 directly without a requirement for complement[18]. The existence of a complement-independent mechanism for binding to macrophages is potentially important for interaction with macrophages in the alveolus, which is considered to be a complement-poor environment[19]. Indeed, in a recent report a fragment of genomic DNA from *M.tb.* was cloned, which confers on non-pathogenic *E. coli* the ability to invade epithelial cells and to enhance their uptake and survival in macrophages, in the absence of complement[20].

These are not esoteric studies. An understanding of the precise mechanism for attachment of *M.tb.* to macrophages will enable us to design new classes of drugs that interfere with this binding, as well as of vaccines that elicit an immune response to these critical surface components of the bacillus.

toxic radicals such as nitric oxide and derivatives[22], antibacterial peptides called defensins[23], and exposure to lysosomes that contain an entire battery of destructive enzymes[24]. Despite these defenses, *M.tb.* is able to establish a chronic infection of macrophages that, in the unactivated state, (see below, *Immune Response*), seem incapable of killing the organism[25,26] (Fig. 2.2). How does the bacillus do it?

An early clue was provided by the now classic electron microscopic study of Armstrong and Hart[27], in which it was shown that live, but not dead, virulent *M.tb.* inhibit fusion of phagosomes and lysosomes, thereby escaping exposure to lysosomal enzymes. In contrast, when tubercle bacilli are opsonized with immune serum prior to phagocytosis, fusion is *not* inhibited[28]. This implies that viable tubercle bacilli actively inhibit phagolysosomal fusion, which at least in part must depend on the specific route of attachment and entry. If this is modified by coating the bacilli with antibody, then presumably phagocytosis occurs via the Fc receptor (which recognizes antibody-coated particles) instead of the complement receptor, thus allowing fusion of phagosomes and lysosomes to occur.

Whereas inhibition of phagolysosomal fusion appears to provide a satisfying answer to the question of how *M.tb.* persists inside macrophages, a problem arose with the observation that the growth of *M.tb.* was identical irrespective of fusion or non-fusion of phagosomes and lysosomes[28]. This does not lessen the significance of inhibition of phagolysosomal fusion in tuberculosis infections,

Internalization of Adherent *M.tb.*

The process of internalization highlights the importance, from a pathogen's perspective, of selecting a particular macrophage receptor as the point of attachment, rather than being engulfed non-specifically. By choosing the CR3, *M.tb.* is internalized by a route that specifically avoids the respiratory burst and release of toxic O_2 radicals that frequently accompanies phagocytosis of bacteria[21]; this is likely to be the reason why attachment and uptake via the CR3 is such a favored route among intracellular macrophage pathogens[14]. In addition, it is likely that the specific use of the CR3 by *M.tb.* also influences the subsequent fate of the internalized organism, as discussed below.

Survival and Growth of Intracellular *M.tb.*

Once inside the macrophage, bacilli have to overcome a formidable array of host defenses, including

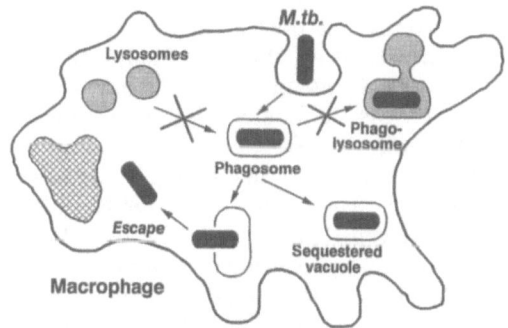

Fig. 2.2. Survival of *M.tb.* within macrophages. After invasion, *M.tb.* has the remarkable capacity for long-term survival and growth within macrophages. The bacilli reside within phagosomes, which resist fusion with toxic lysosomes, preventing conversion of phagosomes into phagolysosomes. Instead, the phagosome is converted into a specialised compartment, or sequestered vacuole, to which normal host defenses do not have access. Alternatively, the bacilli escape from the phagosome and reside freely within the cytoplasm, again removing themselves from toxic host defences.

especially since this is a property of virulent and not avirulent strains of the *M.tb.* complex[29], and is more prominent in macrophages from "susceptible" animals[30] (see below, *Genetics of Host Susceptibility*). It is possible that inhibition of phagolysosomal fusion is important for long-term intracellular survival of virulent *M.tb.* not because of protection from lysosomal enzymes, but rather because this restricts the processing of secreted antigens for presentation to T lymphocytes and thereby dampens the immune response[31].

In addition to inhibition of phagolysosomal fusion, an alternative survival strategy for *M.tb.* might be escape from the phagosome into the cytoplasm, a technique well known among certain intracellular pathogens, such as *L. monocytogenes* and *M. leprae*[14]. Although this exposes the pathogen to other problems (discussed below, *Immune Response*), it does allow the organism to bypass the lysosome completely. Indeed, disruption of the phagosome membrane by *M.tb.* has been observed[29,32], and has recently been bolstered by the detection of cytolytic activity in virulent *M.tb.* which could mediate the disruption of phagosome membranes[33].

M. tuberculosis and the Immune Response

Infection with *M. tuberculosis* presents a dilemma, in terms of understanding the host immune response, that we presently cannot resolve. Whereas it is estimated that one-third of the world's population is *infected* with *M.tb.*, there are "only" 30 million cases of *active disease* in the world today, with 8–10 million new cases annually[34]. Put another way, an individual who is infected with *M.tb.* only has a 5%–10% lifetime risk of developing active tuberculous disease[3]. Thus, purely on epidemiological grounds, we can state emphatically that the great majority of humans develop true *protective* immunity to the disease. However, the dilemma resides in the fact that we can offer no coherent mechanistic explanation for this remarkably effective immune response. All efforts to demonstrate in the laboratory effective killing of tubercle bacilli, or even significant inhibition of growth, by activated human macrophages with or without accessory cells such as T lymphocytes, have failed[25,35,36]. How, then, does the body contain or even eliminate a tuberculous infection? What follows is an account of current attempts to answer this critical question, which has a

profound bearing on the development of new vaccines and other anti-TB strategies.

The Standard Model

First proposed by Mackaness[37], among others, this model suggests that protective immunity is a function of the effective development of delayed type hypersensitivity, which results in activation of infected macrophages and killing of intracellular bacilli. Thus, defense against *M.tb.* is predominantly a cell-mediated immune response, with the following sequence of events. *M.tb.*-containing air-borne droplets are carried into the alveoli of the lungs where the bacilli invade resting alveolar macrophages. The organisms are initially able to grow and multiply unrestrained within the original macrophages, killing these and infecting additional macrophages recruited from blood monocytes. During this phase of unchecked growth, probably lasting 2–4 weeks, the bacilli spread to draining regional lymph nodes and hematogenously throughout the body, infecting tissue macrophages in numerous, distant sites. After 2–4 weeks, however, T-cell-mediated delayed-type hypersensitivity develops as a result of sensitization of T lymphocytes by mycobacterial antigens presented on the surfaces of infected macrophages. These T cells, of the T-helper subset, then secrete cytokines (local hormones) which activate the infected macrophages, enabling them to kill the ingested bacilli. The concerted action of activated macrophages and T cells results in the formation, under the influence of cytokines such as tumor necrosis factor alpha (TNF-α), interferon gamma (INF-γ), and interleukin-2 (IL-2), of well-organized granulomata, which consist of a central area of "caseous" necrosis, surrounding macrophages and epithelioid cells (activated macrophages), and a peripheral cuff of lymphocytes. The growth of *M.tb.* is contained, with eventual organization and fibrosis of the necrotic granulomatous lesion[38].

The Modified Model

The main difficulty with the standard model has been the failure to show that human macrophages, activated or not, can kill *M.tb.*[25,35,36]. The main modification that has been introduced derives from the observation that an important component of the immune response to *M.tb.* is cytotoxic T cells, in addition to T-helper cells and macrophages[10,39–42]. Although originally controversial because cytotoxic T lymphocytes (CTLs) were thought to be primarily involved in defense against viruses and tumor cells, it is now being increasingly accepted that CTLs play an important role in the defense against intracellular bacteria in general, and *M.tb.* in particular[43].

The view that is now emerging is that virulent *M.tb.* are unlikely to be killed by infected macrophages that become activated by sensitized T-helper cells. Instead, infected macrophages are lysed by CTLs with release of bacilli. Lysis of infected macrophages may inhibit or kill *M.tb.* for one of three reasons. First, bacilli may be damaged during the process of cell lysis due to release of lysosomal contents or generation of toxic oxygen or nitrogen radicals[44]. Second, discharge of the bacteria into the centre of caseous necrosis exposes them to an environment not conducive to further growth, due to such factors as low pH and Po_2, and sundry toxic products that may include unsaturated fatty acids and lysophospholipids[43,45]. Third, the released bacteria are now accessible to newly arrived, monocyte-derived macrophages that are highly activated by the abundance of potent cytokines released by infected macrophages, CTLs, and T-helper cells. These activated bystander macrophages are much more able to kill virulent bacilli, probably during the process of phagocytosis, than are the lame and tired, chronically infected macrophages[10,41,44].

In summary, then, the best explanation we now have for protective immunity in TB, is that this depends on a complex and concerted interplay of infected and activated bystander macrophages together with various types of T lymphocytes including cytotoxic and helper cells. These organize into the familiar granuloma with central caseous necrosis (probably comprising lysed macrophages) within which virulent *M.tb.* are contained and perhaps eliminated. Other than pointing to obvious immune deficiencies, such as occur in AIDS, malignancies, or malnutrition, there is at present no general explanation as to why in approximately 5% of individuals this protective immunity breaks down and the bacillus causes overt disease. One of several possible reasons may be the genetic background of the host, as discussed below.

Tuberculosis and HIV Infection

One of the most important factors contributing to the resurgence of TB in the Western world is HIV infection. Dual infections with *M.tb.* and HIV pose a variety of peculiar and often serious problems. Unlike seronegative individuals, who once infected

with *M.tb.* have an approximate 10% lifetime risk of developing active tuberculous disease, in HIV-infected individuals this risk jumps to a 10% *annual* risk[1]. Moreover, disease progression is extremely rapid, sometimes developing within 4 weeks of exposure[46]. Even worse is the observation that the great majority of multidrug-resistant TB occurs in HIV-infected individuals – perhaps as many as 90% of cases – and mortality in these cases approaches 90%, with death ensuing 4–16 weeks after diagnosis[4]. Compounding all of this is the frequent difficulty in diagnosis, because HIV-infected patients are frequently anergic (i.e., unresponsive to a skin test), and TB presents with non-traditional radiographic manifestations[1].

None of this should be particularly surprising, since AIDS by definition is a serious and global immune deficiency state, and it has been known for decades that individuals with depressed immunity – due to such factors as malnutrition, old age, or malignancies – are particularly susceptible to active TB. As is well known, HIV infects and destroys the so-called CD4 lymphocytes, which are the T-helper lymphocytes described in the previous section (*M. tuberculosis and the Immune Response*). Thus the very cells that orchestrate delayed-type hypersensitivity and are vital for the process of macrophage activation (see Figs 2.3 and 2.4) are destroyed by the virus. In addition, there is the suspicion that,

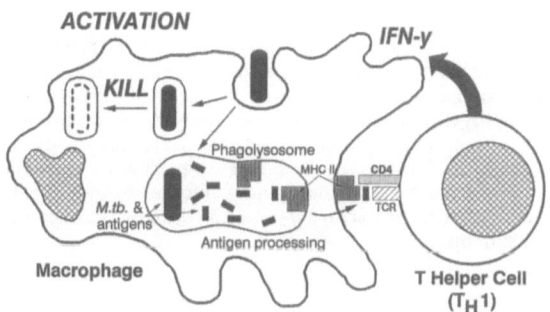

Fig. 2.3. Protective immunity: The Standard Model (Macrophage Activation). Developed by Mackaness (1968) and others, this model emphasises the pre-eminent importance of delayed-type hypersensitivity (DTH), which essentially comprises activation of macrophages by specifically sensitized lymphocytes. Following invasion of macrophages by *M.tb.*, antigens derived from the bacilli within the phagolysosome are processed and presented in association with class II major histocompatibility complex (MHC) proteins on the surface of infected macrophages. There the signal is "read" by T lymphocytes of the T helper subset (specifically T_H1 cells), which are stimulated to release powerful local hormones (cytokines), of which the most important is interferon-gamma (IFN-γ). IFN-γ *activates* the infected macrophages, which then acquire superior mycobactericidal properties and kill the bacilli.

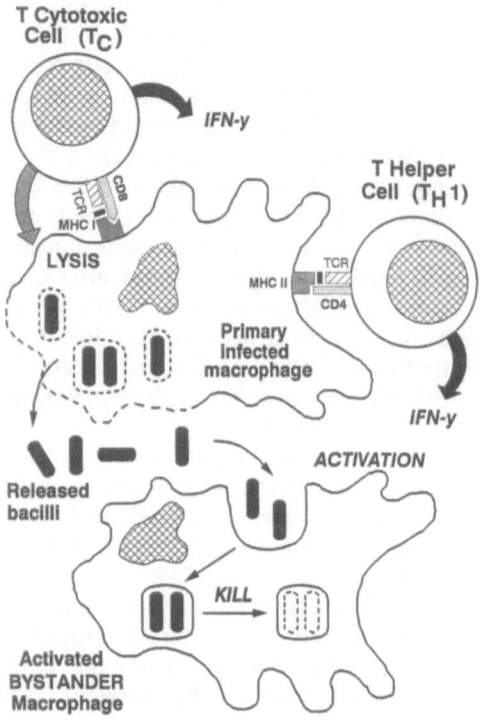

Fig. 2.4. Protective immunity: The Modified Model (Cytolytic Attack and Bystander Killing). Recent research indicates that activation of infected macrophages is by itself not sufficient to control *M.tb.* growth. Instead, what is required is a three-pronged attack comprising T helper cells, T cytotoxic cells, and activated *bystander* macrophages. After invasion, the primary infected macrophages process and present *M.tb.* antigens both in association with class II MHC proteins (for recognition by T helper cells, see Fig. 2.3) and with class I MHC proteins. The latter are recognized by T lymphocytes of the T cytotoxic subset, which promptly lyse (kill) the infected macrophages and release the intracellular bacilli. Both the T helper and T cytotoxic cells produce interferon-gamma (IFN-γ) which activates fresh *bystander* macrophages. These activated macrophages are primed for killing *prior* to ingestion of the released bacilli, and are able to kill the bacilli during or shortly after invasion. Thus the emphasis is shifted from the exhausted primary infected macrophage, to incoming bystander macrophages, which are newly recruited and "fresh for the kill".

not only does HIV infection accelerate the progression of an *M.tb.* infection for the reasons set out above, but infection with *M.tb.*, in turn, accelerates disease progression and the onset of AIDS in an HIV-infected individual. This stems from evidence that latent virus in infected CD4 lymphocytes (i.e. T helper cells) is activated when these same cells are called upon to respond to *M.tb.*-infected macrophages[47]. It is therefore crucial that HIV-positive patients who develop TB are treated as rapidly as possible, and fortunately those seropositive patients with drug-susceptible bacilli usually respond well to anti-tuberculous drugs[4].

Genetics of Host Susceptibility

It has long been suspected that susceptibility to infection with *M. tuberculosis* – and other pathogens, for that matter – is genetically controlled. However, this is also a very controversial view, for a number of reasons. First, although apparent differences in rates of disease have frequently been detected between various racial or ethnic groups and in twin studies[48], it has always been difficult or impossible to assign a clear-cut pattern of inheritance in humans; thus, at the very least, this is likely to be a complex, polygenic trait[49]. Second, there is a large school of thought that regards TB as a social disease and which attributes apparent differences in susceptibility to socio-economic factors; genetic contributions are therefore deemed irrelevant. Third, there is a strong tendency in many quarters to regard with suspicion any attempt to ascribe phenotypic differences of any kind, including disease susceptibility, to racial and genetic differences between population groups. These obstacles notwithstanding, a strong case has been made for the existence of genetic factors in the control of susceptibility to mycobacterial diseases in human populations[48,50].

The *Bcg* Gene

Leaving aside the human studies, impressive evidence has been collected demonstrating that in animals the host response to mycobacteria is genetically determined. In the mouse, the host response to a mycobacterial infection consists of two phases: resistance to the establishment of an infection, sometimes called *innate* resistance; and emergence of protective immunity that controls or eliminates an established infection[49,51]. Both phases are under distinct and separate elements of genetic control, of which the former has been extensively characterized. Studies in mice have revealed that innate resistance to infection by *M. bovis* BCG is controlled by a single autosomal-dominant gene, the *Bcg* gene, located on chromosome 1. Moreover, the *Bcg* gene is either identical or tightly linked to the *Ity* and *Lsh* genes that control resistance to the antigenically unrelated organisms *Salmonella typhimurium* and *Leishmania donovani*, respectively. This has led to the provocative conclusion that a single gene may control resistance to diverse intracellular pathogens (reviewed in refs. 49,51,52). Further studies have strongly implicated the macrophage as the cell in which this gene is expressed and have indicated that the difference in macrophages derived from *Bcg*^r (resistant) mice compared to *Bcg*^s (susceptible) mice resides in a heightened state of activation of the former. Thus, macrophages from Bcg^r mice express superior bactericidal activity and an enhanced capacity to restrict the growth of intracellular pathogens[49].

A candidate for the Bcg gene has been isolated and designated $Nramp$ (for natural resistance-associated macrophage protein)[52]. $Nramp$ encodes a protein that is expressed exclusively in macrophages and which is similar to a family of membrane-associated transport proteins[52]. It has been speculated that the $Nramp$ protein allows nitric oxide (NO) to be concentrated within phagosomes that house $M.tb$; nitric oxide is known to be strongly mycobactericidal[22].

This is clearly an advance of fundamental importance in our understanding of components of the host response to $M.tb$. A homolog of the mouse $Nramp$ gene has been found in the human genome[52], and it remains to be established whether this plays a role in human susceptibility to a tuberculous infection. The implications of finding a TB resistance gene in human populations are enormous for the design of powerful new drugs and vaccines.

Genetics of Protective Immunity

In contrast to work on innate resistance and the Bcg gene, the genetics of protective immunity are much less well defined. There has been an understandable inclination to search for a link between genes for histocompatibility antigens (called MHC genes in the mouse and HLA genes in humans) because of the central importance of these proteins in regulating the manner in which foreign antigens are recognised by T lymphocytes, thought to be the mediators of protective immunity in TB (see earlier)[49]. These studies have indeed met with some success, and in both mice and humans histocompatibility genes do show some association with the development of protective immunity, although this is not as yet clear cut[51].

Vaccines and other Immunomodulatory Strategies

Vaccines are intended to induce a state of protective immunity prior to exposure to a particular virulent pathogen and thereby to prevent clinical disease. As there is little doubt that the majority of individuals infected with $M.tb$. are able to mount an effective protective immune response, with suppression and perhaps even elimination of the infecting bacilli (see earlier), the development of an effective vaccine would seem to be an attainable goal (in contrast, for instance, to the design of an AIDS vaccine, which *a priori* is much more problematic). Having said that, however, the only TB vaccine in clinical use, BCG, is of questionable efficacy and is largely ineffective in preventing the predominant adult form of the disease, post-primary pulmonary TB[53]. There is thus a clear need for a superior vaccine that can reliably offer protection. In addition to a new "conventional" vaccine, we should also consider the introduction of immunomodulatory therapies aimed at tilting the balance from overt disease to effective endogenous protective immunity. This could be considered an adjunct to chemotherapy in patients with established TB.

BCG

The vaccine strain bacillus Calmette–Guérin is named after the researchers who attenuated a virulent strain of *M. bovis* by serial passage in a bizarre artificial medium (potato dipped in bile) between the years 1908 and 1918 in France[53]. Introduced in the 1920s, the vaccine has since been the subject of numerous controlled trials which, almost inexplicably, demonstrate a protective efficacy ranging from nil (or even detrimental) to 80%[53,54]. A variety of quite involved arguments have been invoked to account for this discrepancy, of which perhaps the most convincing is that BCG is primarily or only effective in preventing hematogenous dissemination of bacilli (bacillemia) during the primary infection and not in preventing the growth of localized foci during re-infection or reactivation disease[53,54]. This is consistent with the observation that BCG is most reliable in preventing meningitis and miliary TB, both the result of hematogenously disseminated primary infection. Despite these doubts about this efficacy, BCG continues to be administered worldwide (although with some notable exceptions, including the USA); indeed, it is the most widely used vaccine in the world, with some 3 billion doses administered since its introduction[53]. Continued use is no doubt due to the evidence for limited efficacy ("better than nothing") and to its remarkable safety (case fatality rate of only 0.19 per million[55]).

New TB Vaccines

Given that BCG is problematic, what alternatives might there be? Although various alternatives have been suggested (see below), the primary difficulty currently is that we have no clear concept of what is required to generate true protective immunity. Thus we cannot explain at present in precise molecular terms why BCG is largely ineffective; on the face of it, BCG should be an ideal vaccine, as it is a live, attenuated strain very closely related to *M.tb.*, and it is similarly able to take up an intracellular residence in macrophages[29,54]. It may be argued that BCG lacks one or more critical antigens unique to *M.tb.*[56], or that BCG is unable to persist within macrophages and/or escape into the cytoplasm as virulent strains of *M.tb.* are able to[29]. Once these difficulties have been resolved, the rational design of an alternative vaccine can be undertaken, which could include:

1. *Recombinant BCG.* Depending on which determinants are found to be indispensable to elicit a protective response, these could be engineered into a recombinant BCG vaccine. Indeed, the genetic manipulation of BCG for use as an all-purpose recombinant vaccine is actively in progress[55,57].

2. *Subunit vaccines.* Instead of administering an entire, attenuated, live organism, some have argued in favor of the selective administration of individual immunodominant antigens. This approach depends on the identification of one or more immunodominant antigens that can elicit a protective response. One such immunodominant antigens is the so-called 65-kD protein. This is one of the major secreted proteins of *M.tb.*[58] and was found to be the target of approximately 20% of mycobacteria-reactive T cells in mice that were immunized with *M.tb.*[59]. However, hopes that the 65-kD protein could be used as a recombinant subunit vaccine were dashed by the failure to elicit protective immunity in animal models[56].

3. *Other mycobacteria.* There have been calls for the use of mycobacteria unrelated to the *M.tb.* complex as vaccines. This relates to the observation that variable and complex patterns of protection are apparently elicited by exposure to environmental (generally non-pathogenic) mycobacteria, and this is strongly dependent on geographical location[60]. There is some evidence that administration of a fast-growing environmental mycobacterial strain together with BCG (a slow grower) may synergize in producing a protective response[60] and on the basis of this trials are currently underway to evaluate the usefulness of the environmental strain *M. vaccae.*

Unconventional Immunomodulatory Strategies

The benefits resulting from understanding the mechanism of protective immunity with greater precision will include not only the design of better vaccines for the prevention of disease but also the use of immunomodulatory strategies in the treatment of established TB. This approach is presently still firmly in the realm of experimentation and hypothesis, but a number of possibilities can be entertained.

1. *Augmenting a favourable T-helper response.* As discussed in the section *M. Tuberculosis and the Immune Response* (above), protective immunity depends on the stimulation of T-helper cells that activate macrophages. Macrophage activation is part of the familiar delayed-type hypersensitivity reaction (DTH) which is vital in defense against intracellular pathogens. Recent research has indicated that some T-helper cells promote DTH (called T_H1 cells), whereas others stimulate antibody production (T_H2 cells); moreover one or the other tend to predominate[61]. It is possible that in active tuberculosis a shift has occurred from a favourable T_H1 response to an unfavourable T_H2 response[43]. Restoration of T_H1 cell predominance could become an important therapeutic option in TB.

2. *Therapeutic activation of macrophages.* As was discussed in the section *Genetics of Host Susceptibility*, mice positive for the *Bcg* gene (*Bcg*[r] mice) can substantially restrict the establishment of an infection, and this is thought to be due to a state of inherent or constitutive activation of their macrophages. This may also be true in humans, and a means to generally activate macrophages may represent a powerful preventive and therapeutic approach.

3. *Enhancing cytolytic activity.* The importance of cytotoxic T lymphocytes (CTLs) in protection against *M.tb.* is no longer in doubt[62]. Enhancing CTL activity in individuals unable to control an *M.tb.* infection may, therefore, be useful. Methods for achieving this fall outside the scope of this chapter, but interested readers are referred to the recent review by Lanzavecchia[63]. One caveat that applies to this approach, and for that matter to any form of immunomodulation, is that one may do more harm than good. We do not at present understand the origin of the severe tissue destruction seen in cavitary pulmonary TB, but if this results from an exaggerated cell-mediated immune response (i.e., DTH)

as many believe[41], then further augmentation of macrophage activation and cytolytic activity may seriously aggravate the pathology.

Mechanisms of Drug Resistance

The evolution of multidrug-resistant strains of M.tb. (MDR-TB) is the most sinister recent development in the TB saga and greatly exacerbates the litany of lost opportunities in the world-wide control of this disease. It is further aggravated by the fertile ground offered to the organism by the legions of HIV-infected individuals throughout the world, and it comes as no surprise that MDR-TB is above all a problem in AIDS patients. In these patients, the mortality approaches 90% and death often ensues within 4 weeks of the diagnosis of MDR-TB[1]. The scale of the problem can be appreciated when it is realized that in New York, 34% of new cases of TB are resistant to at least one drug, and fully 19% are resistant to two or more drugs (MDR-TB)[1]. This being such a serious problem – one that could catapult us back to the pre-antibiotic, sanatorium era of TB control[64] – a world-wide effort has been engendered that is aimed at early diagnosis of MDR-TB in clinical isolates, as well as comprehensive basic research into the mechanisms of drug resistance[1,3,12].

Resistance in M.tb. usually results from one or more mutations in the bacterial chromosome[65]. This type of resistance is consistent with the rates of emergence of resistant strains, which are in the order of 10^{-7} to 10^{-8} for most of the major antibiotics, including INH, rifampicin, ethionamide, and streptomycin[65-68]. Frequencies in this order are typical of "single-step" high-level resistance patterns in which resistance is conferred by a single mutation which arises spontaneously in a population of bacteria not previously exposed to the antibiotic[65]. Since cavitatory lung lesions contain in excess of 10^{9} bacilli, the importance of using at least two antituberculous agents can be readily appreciated, since the use of only one antibiotic will rapidly select for pre-existing, spontaneously resistant bacilli in that population[65].

Isoniazid (INH) Resistance

INH is thought to act via the inhibition of the synthesis of mycolic acids, which are an integral part of the mycobacterial cell wall. Two resistance mechan-

isms have been identified to date. The first is unusual in that it is due to the deletion of the katG gene that codes for both catalase and peroxidase in mycobacteria[69]. It is likely that the katG gene is required for the antimycobacterial activity of INH and that its deletion renders the drug inactive[69]. The second resistance mechanism is more conventional. A single missense mutation has been found in a gene designated inhA, which encodes a protein that is strongly homologous to enzymes involved in fatty acid synthesis (mycolic acid is a type of fatty acid)[68]. Thus, here we have an example of a single chromosomal mutation conferring resistance. The inhA mutation also confers resistance to ethionamide, a structural analog of INH[68].

Rifampicin Resistance

Rifampicin inhibits the bacterial RNA polymerase, and in other bacteria resistance is due to specific mutations in the gene coding for RNA polymerase subunit β (the rpoB gene). A similar mechanism has now also been shown for M.tb. In 64 of 66 rifampicin-resistant isolates, mutations involving 8 conserved amino acids were found, all clustered within a region of 23 amino acids on the rpoB gene[66]. Thus, rifampicin resistance is conferred by one of a number of single-step mutations within a small stretch of DNA of the rpoB gene in M.tb.

Streptomycin Resistance

In common with all aminoglycoside antibiotics, streptomycin inhibits bacterial protein synthesis by binding to the 30S ribosomal subunit. The ribosomal S12 protein is part of the 30S subunit and a point mutation conferring streptomycin resistance has been found in the rpsL gene encoding the S12 protein in a number of M.tb. strains[67].

Multidrug-resistant (MDR)-TB

Available clinical and epidemiological data are consistent with the notion that MDR-TB strains can arise by sequential accumulation of resistance mechanisms for individual drugs. In addition it is possible, although there is presently no direct evidence, that multidrug resistance could result from a generalized mechanism such as an efficient drug-degradation system, increased permeability barrier to multiple drugs, or over-expression of a drug export pump[67].

Early Detection of MDR-TB

Many patients with MDR-TB die before the results of drug susceptibility testing become available; this delay also exposes associated health-care workers to serious risks[1,66]. Clearly there is an urgent need for a rapid and facile method for susceptibility testing that improves on the 6–8 weeks required for the present standard methods. Two innovative methods that have been proposed are worth discussion:

1. *Genetic testing for drug resistance mutations.* As the genetic basis for drug resistance is being elucidated, rapid PCR-based methods can be developed that allow detection of particular mutations. This has been suggested for the rifampicin-resistance mutations, which as elaborated above, are clustered within a small region of the *rpoB* gene[66]. Since rifampicin resistance is present in most isolates of MDR-TB[1], this could be a useful surrogate marker for MDR-TB[66].

2. *Luciferase reporter phages.* An ingenious alternative is the infection of *M.tb.* with a mycobacteriophage engineered to express the firefly luciferase gene. In bacilli that are viable and contain adequate quantities of ATP, light is produced, whereas in those that are inhibited or dying, light production is extinguished[70]. Once an adequate culture of *M.tb.* has been obtained from a clinical isolate, the use of luciferase reporter phages could reduce the time required for antibiotic sensitivity testing from weeks to hours.

Prospects for New Developments

The study of mycobacteria has entered the era of molecular biology and has been radically transformed, as has virtually every area of biomedical research. Moreover, the alarming resurgence of TB in the Western world and the sinister menace of MDR-TB have galvanized public health officials, increased funding and prestige associated with mycobacterial research, and consequently have encouraged a new breed of molecular microbiologists to attack, once again, this age-old scourge. This chapter has highlighted some of the early fruits of these recent endeavors and indicated areas of active research. There is no doubt that we are standing at the threshold of making incisive advances in our attempts to contain this disease. The fundamental breakthroughs which are being, and have been, made in the mechanisms of invasion and survival in macrophages, and in the critical elements of the protective immune response, will enable the rational design of new therapeutic and preventive strategies. The cornerstone has been laid for the development of the armamentarium required finally and irrevocably – albeit many decades hence – to close the book on this terrible disease.

References

1. Ellner JJ, Hinman AR, Dooley SW, Fischl MA, Sepkowitz KA, Goldberger MJ, Shinnick TM, Iseman MD, Jacobs Jr. WR (1993) Tuberculosis symposium: emerging problems and promise. J Infect Dis 168: 537–551
2. Centers for Disease Control (1989) A strategic plan for the elimination of tuberculosis in the United States. MMWR 38 (suppl. S-3): 1–25
3. Bloom BR, Murray CJL (1992) Tuberculosis: commentary on a reemergent killer. Science 257: 1055–1064
4. Snider Jr. DE, Roper WL (1992) The new tuberculosis. N Engl J Med 326: 703–705
5. Ehlers MRW (1993) The wolf at the door. Some thoughts on the biochemistry of the tubercle bacillus. S Afr Med J 82: 900–903
6. Goodfellow M, Wayne LG (1982) Taxonomy and nomenclature. In: Ratledge C, Stanford JL (eds.) The Biology of the Mycobacteria, vol 1. London: Academic Press, pp 471–521
7. McNeil MR, Brennan PJ (1991) Structure, function and biogenesis of the cell envelope of mycobacteria in relation to bacterial physiology, pathogenesis and drug resistance; some thoughts and possibilities arising from recent structural information. Res. Microbiol. 142, 451–463
8. Young DB, Kaufmann SHE, Hermans PWM, Thole JER (1992) Mycobacterial protein antigens: a compilation. Mol Microbiol 6: 133–145
9. Barnes PF, Mehra V, Hirschfield GR, Fong S-J, Abou-Zeid C, Rook GAW, Hunter SW, Brennan PJ, Modlin RL (1989) Characterization of T cell antigens associated with the cell wall protein-peptidoglycan complex of *Mycobacterium tuberculosis*. J Immunol 143: 2656–2662
10. Orme IA, Miller ES, Roberts AD, Furney SK, Griffin JP, Dobos KM, Chi D, Rivoire B, Brennan PJ (1992) T lymphocytes mediating protection and cellular cytolysis during the course of *Mycobacterium tuberculosis* infection. Evidence for different kinetics and recognition of a wide spectrum of protein antigens. J Immunol 148: 189–196
11. North RJ, Izzo AA (1993) Mycobacterial virulence. Virulent strains of *Mycobacterium tuberculosis* have faster in vivo doubling times and are better equipped to resist growth-inhibiting functions of macrophages in the presence and absence of specific immunity. J Exp Med 177: 1723–1733
12. Young DB, Cole ST (1993) Minireview. Leprosy, tuberculosis, and the New Genetics. J Bact 175: 1–6
13. Nyka W (1974) Studies on the effect of starvation on mycobacteria. Infect Immun 9: 843–850
14. Falkow S, Isberg RR, Portnoy DA (1992) The interaction of bacteria with mammalian cells. Annu Rev Cell Biol 8: 333–363
15. Schlesinger LS, Bellinger-Kawahara CG, Payne NR, Horwitz MA (1990) Phagocytosis of *Mycobacterium tuberculosis* is

mediated by human monocyte complement receptors and complement component C3. J Immunol 144: 2771–2780

16. Hynes RO (1992) Integrins: versatility, modulation, and signalling in cell adhesion. Cell 69: 11–25

17. Bliska JB, Galán JE, Falkow S (1993) Signal transduction in the mammalian cell during bacterial attachment and entry. Cell 73: 903–920

18. Isberg RR, Van Nhieu GT (1994) Binding and internalization of microorganisms by integrin receptors. Trends Microbiol 2: 10–14

19. Ofek I, Rest RF, Sharon N (1992) Nonopsonic phagocytosis of microorganisms. Phagocytes use several molecular mechanisms to recognize, bind, and eventually kill microorganisms. ASM News 58: 429–435

20. Arruda S, Bomfim G, Knights R, Huima-Byron T, Riley LW (1993) Cloning of an M. tuberculosis DNA fragment associated with entry and survival inside cells. Science 261: 1454–1457

21. Wright SD, Silverstein SC (1983) Receptors for C3b and C3bi promote phagocytosis but not the release of toxic oxygen from human phagocytes. J Exp Med 158: 2016–2023

22. Chan J, Xing Y, Magliozzo RS, Bloom BR (1992) Killing of virulent Mycobacterium tuberculosis by reactive nitrogen intermediates produced by activated murine macrophages. J Exp Med 175: 1111–1122

23. Lehrer RI, Ganz T, Selsted ME (1991) Defensins: endogenous antibiotic peptides of animal cells. Cell 64: 229–230

24. Auger MJ, Ross JA (1992) The biology of the macrophage. In: Lewis CE, McGee, J O'D (eds) The Macrophage. Oxford: IRL Press, pp 1–74

25. Rook GAW (1988) Role of activated macrophages in the immunopathology of tuberculosis. Br Med Bull 44: 611–623

26. Lowrie DB, Andrew PW (1988) Macrophage antimycobacterial mechanisms. Br Med Bull 44: 624–634

27. Armstrong JA, Hart P D'Arcy (1971) Response of cultured macrophages to Mycobacterium tuberculosis, with observations on fusion of lysosomes with phagosomes. J Exp Med 134: 713–740

28. Armstrong JA, Hart P D'Arcy (1975) Phagosome-lysosome interactions in cultured macrophages infected with virulent tubercle bacilli. J Exp Med 142: 1–16

29. McDonough KA, Kress Y, Bloom BR (1993) Pathogenesis of tuberculosis: interaction of Mycobacterium tuberculosis with macrophages. Infect Immun 61: 2763–2773

30. De Chastellier C, Fréhel C, Offredo C, Skamene E. (1993) Implication of phagosome-lysosome fusion in restriction of Mycobacterium avium growth in bone marrow macrophages from genetically resistant mice. Infect Immun 61: 3775–3784

31. Pancholi P, Mirza A, Bhardwaj N, Steinman RM (1993) Sequestration from immune CD4+ T cells of mycobacteria growing in human macrophages. Science 260: 984–986

32. Myrvik QN, Leake ES, Wright MJ (1984) Disruption of phagosomal membranes of normal alveolar macrophages by the H37Rv strain of Mycobacterium tuberculosis. Am Rev Respir Dis 129: 322–328

33. King CH, Mundayoor S, Crawford JT, Shinnick TM (1993) Expression of contact-dependent cytolytic activity by Mycobacterium tuberculosis and isolation of the genomic locus that encodes the activity. Infect Immun 61: 2708–2712

34. Friedman H, Bendinelli M (1988) Preface. In: Bendinelli M, Friedman H (eds) Mycobacterium tuberculosis. Interactions with the Immune System. New York: Plenum Press, pp xi–xiii.

35. Rook GAW, Steele J, Ainsworth M, Champion BR (1986) Activation of macrophages to inhibit proliferation of Mycobacterium tuberculosis: comparison of the effects of

36. Collins FM (1990) In vivo vs. in vitro killing of virulent Mycobacterium tuberculosis. Res Microbiol 141: 212–217

37. Mackaness GB (1968) The immunology of antituberculous immunity. Am Rev Resp Dis 97: 337–344

38. Lucas SB (1989) Mycobacteria and the tissues of man. In: Ratledge C, Stanford J, Grange JM (eds) The Biology of the Mycobacteria vol. 3. London: Academic Press, pp 107–176

39. De Libero G, Flesch I, Kaufmann SHE (1988) Mycobacteria-reactive Lyt-2+ T cell lines. Eur J Immunol 18: 59–66

40. Ottenhoff THM, Ab BK, Van Embden JDA, Thole JER, Kiessling R (1988) The recombinant 65-kD heat shock protein of Mycobacterium bovis bacillus Calmette-Guerin/M. tuberculosis is a target molecule for CD4+ cytotoxic T lymphocytes that lyse human monocytes. J Exp Med 168: 1947–1952

41. Pithie AD, Rahelu M, Kumararatne DS, Drysdale P, Gaston JSH, Iles PB, Innes JA, Ellis CJ (1992) Generation of cytolytic T cells in individuals infected by Mycobacterium tuberculosis and vaccinated with BCG. Thorax 47: 695–701

42. Flynn JL, Goldstein MM, Triebold KJ, Koller B, Bloom BR (1992) Major histocompatibility complex class I-restricted T cells are required for resistance to Mycobacterium tuberculosis infection. Proc Natl Acad Sci USA 89: 12013–12017

43. Kaufmann SHE (1993) Immunity to intracellular bacteria. Annu Rev Immunol 11: 129–163

44. Kaufmann SHE, De Libero G (1988) Cytolytic cells in M. tuberculosis infections. In: Bendinelli M, Friedman H (eds) Mycobacterium tuberculosis. Interactions with the Immune System. New York: Plenum Press, pp 151–170

45. Lowrie DB (1983) Mononuclear phagocyte-mycobacterium interaction. In: Ratledge C, Stanford J (eds) The Biology of the Mycobacteria vol. 2, London: Academic Press, pp 235–278

46. Daley CL, Small PM, Schecter GF, Schoolnik GK, McAdam RA, Jacobs Jr. WR, Hopewell PC (1992). An outbreak of tuberculosis with accelerated progression among persons infected with the human immunodeficiency virus. N Engl J Med 326: 231–235

47. Hannibal MC, Markovitz DM, Clark N, Nabel GJ (1993) Differential activation of human immunodeficiency virus type 1 and 2 transcription by specific T-cell activation signals. J Virol 67: 5035–5040

48. Stead WW (1992) Genetics and resistance to tuberculosis: could resistance be enhanced by genetic engineering? Ann Intern Med 116: 937–941

49. Buschman E, Skamene E (1988) Genetic background of the host and expression of natural resistance and acquired immunity to M. tuberculosis. In: Bendinelli M, Friedman H (eds) Mycobacterium tuberculosis. Interactions with the Immune System. New York: Plenum Press, pp 59–79

50. Schurr E, Morgan K, Gros P, Skamene E (1991) Genetics of leprosy. Am J Trop Med Hyg 44: 4–11

51. Buschman E, Schurr E, Gros P, Skamene E (1990) Role of major histocompatibility complex (MHC) and non-MHC genes in host resistance and susceptibility to mycobacteria. In: Ayoub EM, Cassell GH, Branche Jr. WC, Henry TJ (eds) American Society for Microbiology, Microbial Determinants of Virulence and Host Response. Washington, D.C: pp 93–111

52. Vidal SM, Malo D, Vogan K, Skamene E, Gros P (1993) Natural resistance to infection with intracellular parasites: isolation of a candidate for Bcg. Cell 73: 469–485

53. Fine PEM, Rodrigues LC (1990) Modern vaccines. Mycobacterial diseases. Lancet 335: 1016–1020

54. Smith DW, Wiegeshaus EH, Edwards ML (1988) The protective effects of BCG vaccination against tuberculosis. In: Bendinelli M, Friedman H, (eds) Mycobacterium tuberculo-

sis. Interaction with the Immune System. New York: Plenum Press, pp 341–370

55. Stover CK, de la Cruz VF, Fuerst TR, Burlein JE, Benson LA, Bennett LT, Bansal GP, Young JF, Lee MH, Hatfull GF, Snapper SB, Barletta RG, Jacobs Jr. WR, Bloom BR (1991) New use of BCG for recombinant vaccines. Nature 351: 456–460

56. Colston MJ (1990) Protective immunity against mycobacterial infections: investigating cloned antigens. In: McFadden J (ed) Molecular Biology of the Mycobacteria. London: Surrey University Press, pp 69–76

57. Aldovini A, Young RA (1991) Humoral and cell-mediated immune responses to live recombinant BCG-HIV vaccines. Nature 351: 479–482

58. Young D, Garbe T, Lathigra R, Abou-Zeid C (1990) Protein antigens: structure, function and regulation. In: McFadden J (ed) Molecular Biology of the Mycobacteria. London: Surrey University Press, pp 1–35

59. Kaufmann SHE, Vath U, Thole JER, van Embden JDA, Emmrich F (1987) Enumeration of T cells reactive with *Mycobacterium tuberculosis* organisms and specific for the recombinant mycobacterial 64-kDa protein. Eur J Immunol 17: 351–357

60. Shield MJ (1983) The importance of immunologically effective contact with environmental mycobateria. In: Ratledge C, Stanford J (eds) The Biology of the Mycobacteria, vol. 2. London: Academic Press, pp 343–415

61. Paul WE, Seder RA (1994) Lymphocyte responses and cytokines. Cell 76: 241–251

62. Ehlers S, Mielke MEA, Hahn H (1994) Progress in TB research: Robert Koch's dilemma revisited. Immunol. Today 15, 1–4

63. Lanzavecchia A (1993) Identifying strategies for immune intervention. Science 260: 937–944

64. Bloom BR (1992) Tuberculosis. Back to a frightening future. Nature 358: 538–539

65. Mitchison DA (1984) Drug resistance in mycobacteria. Br Med Bull 40: 84–90

66. Telenti A, Imboden P, Marchesi F, Lowrie D, Cole S, Colston MJ, Matter L, Schopfer K, Bodmer T (1993) Detection of rifampicin-resistance mutations in *Mycobacterium tuberculosis.* Lancet 341: 647–650

67. Nair J, Rouse DA, Bai G-H, Morris SL (1993) The *rpsL* gene and streptomycin resistance in single and multiple drug-resistant strains of *Mycobacterium tuberculosis.* Mol Microbiol 10: 521–527

68. Banerjee A, Dubnau E, Quemard A, Balasubramanian V, Um KS, Wilson T, Collins D, de Lisle G, Jacobs Jr. WR (1994) *inhA,* a gene encoding a target for isoniazid and ethionamide in *Mycobacterium tuberculosis.* Science 263: 227–230

69. Zhang Y, Heym B, Allen B, Young D, Cole S (1992) The catalase-peroxidase gene and isoniazid resistance of *Mycobacterium tuberculosis.* Nature 358: 591–593

70. Jacobs Jr. WR, Barletta RG, Udani R, Chan J, Kalkut G, Sosne G, Kieser T, Sarkis GJ, Hatfull GF, Bloom BR (1993) Rapid assessment of drug susceptibilities of *Mycobacterium tuberculosis* by means of luciferase reporter phages. Science 260: 819–822

3 Imaging of Pulmonary Tuberculosis

B.J. Cremin and D.H. Jamieson

Imaging Methods

1. *Conventional*
   a. *Chest X-ray* (CXR) is the most cost-effective modality for the initial evaluation and follow-up. Frontal and lateral CXRs are required for adequate assessment. Films in non-rotation, full inspiration and with sufficient penetration to show at least the upper thoracic vertebrae are required.
   b. *Mass miniatures* have been largely abandoned because of a low yield in early cases[1,2].
   c. *High kV filtered X-rays* are useful for demonstrating both extrinsic compression and intrinsic involvement of trachea and main bronchi by mediastinal adenopathy. The CXR in children is often well penetrated so that filtration is recommended for high kV films to block out the softer "bone seeking" X-rays, reduce scatter and harden the beam. A filter of 0.4-mm tin, 0.5-mm copper and 0.75-mm aluminum in the collimator has been recommended[3]. Our adaptation is a 1-mm copper, 1-mm aluminum filter and use of a fluoroscopy table for positioning and increasing the patient to film distance to produce some magnification.
   d. *Bronchography* has largely fallen into abeyance and been replaced by high resolution computed tomography (HRCT) since the non-availability of suitable oily bronchographic agents. The advantage of an oily contrast medium was that a 24 h film showed pathological retention of contrast medium in affected bronchi, providing evidence of inability to clear secretions.

2. *Digital Radiography*
   Digital radiography is superior to plain radiography for evaluation of soft tissues and adenopathy. It is not universally available but one can make use of the routine survey study from CT scans.

3. *Computed Tomography (CT)*
   Computed tomography very useful to evaluate mediastinal, parenchymal, pleural and pericardial pathology. It is an important modality for problem solving when CXR is equivocal. One of its main uses is to demonstrate adenopathy by dynamic contrast studies which are performed by taking 0.5–1-cm slices in a dynamic mode during the injection of contrast medium in a dosage up to 4 ml/kg of a 300 mg/ml iodine contrast agent. Sedation is essential in young children and 100–150 mg/kg of chloral hydrate up to 2 g is usually satisfactory. CT is useful to demonstrate occult cavitation, evaluate nodular interstitial disease and define the extent of bronchiectasis. High resolution computed tomography (HRCT) techniques using limited thin slices (1–2 mm) and edge enhancing reconstruction algorithms are helpful in assessing both bronchial and parenchymal disease. Pericardial and pleural effusion can be accurately assessed and when ultrasound (US) access is poor, CT is particularly useful in localizing the extent of pleural collections prior to drainage.

4. *Magnetic Resonance Imaging (MR)*
   Magnetic resonance imaging has similar uses to CT but cost and lack of availability restrict its use. It is very effective in demonstrating adenopathy both because of its multiplanar imaging capacity and because it allows ready identification of vessels due to their flow void characteristics. For optimum use cardiac gating and fast acquisition techniques are required.

5. *Ultrasound (US)*

    Ultrasound is a useful modality to assess pleural and pericardial effusions. It is also helpful for detecting paratracheal adenopathy and distinguishing it from normal thymus using a parasternal or supraclavicular approach.

6. *Isotopes*

    Isotopes are not used in routine studies but are useful if a preoperative assessment of lung function is required.

The assessment of primary pulmonary TB is best understood by considering it as the initial infection with a primary complex, subsequent development of lymphobronchial disease with its complications, disseminated disease and late parenchymal pathology.

There can be no routine description of TB chest lesions, particularly in children with deficient immunity. The protean nature of the reaction to infection does not lead to any universally expected appearance[4] and TB may produce almost any form of CXR abnormality[5]. However, there are common radiographic patterns, and the following appearances in a child should alert us to the diagnosis. These include:

1. Enlarged mediastinal or hilar lymph nodes with or without parenchymal lesions (Figs 3.1, 3.2, 3.3).

2. Persistent chest pathology that does not respond to routine antibiotics. This particularly applies to right middle lobe (RML) pathology, as the RML bronchus is susceptible to nodal compression (Fig. 3.4).

3. The rapid and unexplained appearance of a nodular reticular pattern (Fig. 3.5a, b).

4. Finally a review of a series of CXRs may be the most important factor in establishing a diagnosis of TB.

Initial Infection – Primary Complex

The initial pneumonic reaction to infection in the lung is the Ghon focus[6]. The combination of the initial inflammatory pulmonary focus and lymphangitic spread to involve regional lymph nodes constitutes the primary complex or Rankes complex[7] (Fig. 3.6) A Ghon focus may occur anywhere in the lung and may be multiple in at least 25% of cases[8]

(Fig. 3.7). The focus is usually small and round but may enlarge so that it may be difficult to differentiate from the segmental lesion of lymphobronchial disease[9] (Fig. 3.8). In a Nigerian study, 47 of 273 cases (17%) were reported as having a primary complex[10] but the authors' experience is that identification of a true primary complex is not common in asymptomatic children. The relatively insidious nature of the primary infection, with its non-specific constitutional symptoms, accounts for its presentation to hospital only when complications have developed. The lymph node enlargement is prominent, usually unilateral and persists longer than the parenchymal lesion. During the healing process nodes and parenchymal lesions may calcify (Fig. 3.9).

When the lesion persists or spreads to become progressive primary disease, the spectrum enlarges into lymphobronchial disease with segmental lesions, previously known as endobronchial TB or epituberculosis[11]. This results in varying degrees of segmental or lobar consolidation, cavitation and collapse or over-expansion, all of which can be visualized by both conventional radiology and modern imaging techniques.

Adenopathy

Hilar and mediastinal lymphadenopathy is the radiographic hallmark of primary TB. The reported incidence of adenopathy seen on CXR varies from 63%[9,10] to 95%[12,13,14]. Adenopathy is more frequently seen in the younger child (<3 years) and overall recognition of adenopathy as an early sign at this age is about 85%.

A normal CXR does not exclude TB and may correspond to minimal active disease rather than absence of disease[15]. A study of 185 cases of bacteriologically proven TB cases in the Western Cape of South Africa had only 3 normal CXRs (1.6%), all of which subsequently developed abnormalities[9]. A recent Canadian study had a higher incidence with 14 out of 191 cases initially reported as normal (7%)[12].

The presence of pulmonary pathology without adenopathy makes the radiological diagnosis difficult (Fig. 3.10). However the persistence of consolidation following adequate antibiotic treatment must raise the suspicion of TB, and the use of contrast enhanced CT increases the detection of lymph nodes, which may be obscured by lung or pleural pathology.

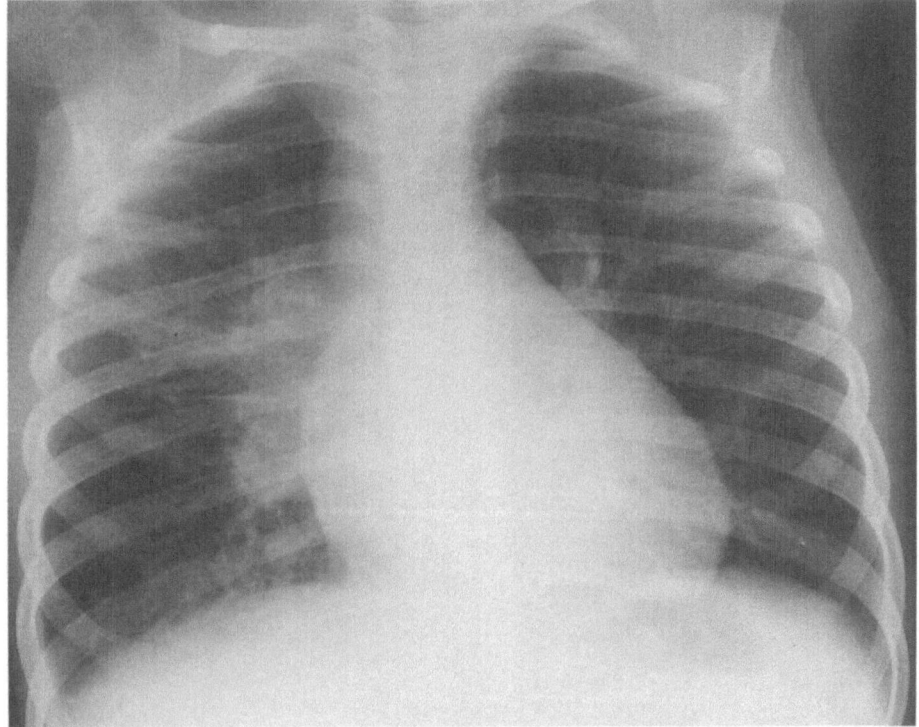

a

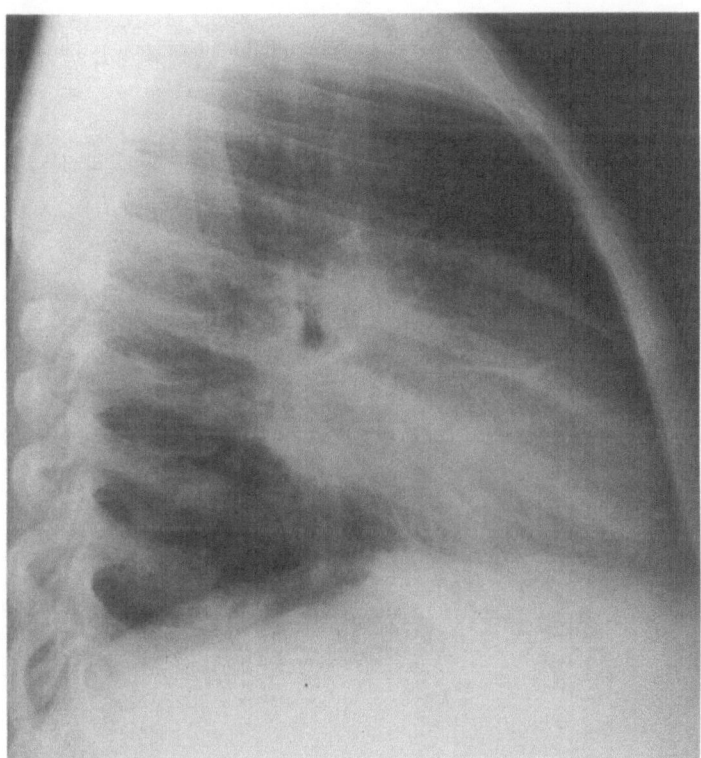

b

Fig. 3.1a, b. CXR AP and lateral; prominent R hilar and R paratracheal adenopathy with parenchymal infiltrate in the RUL is typical of primary TB.

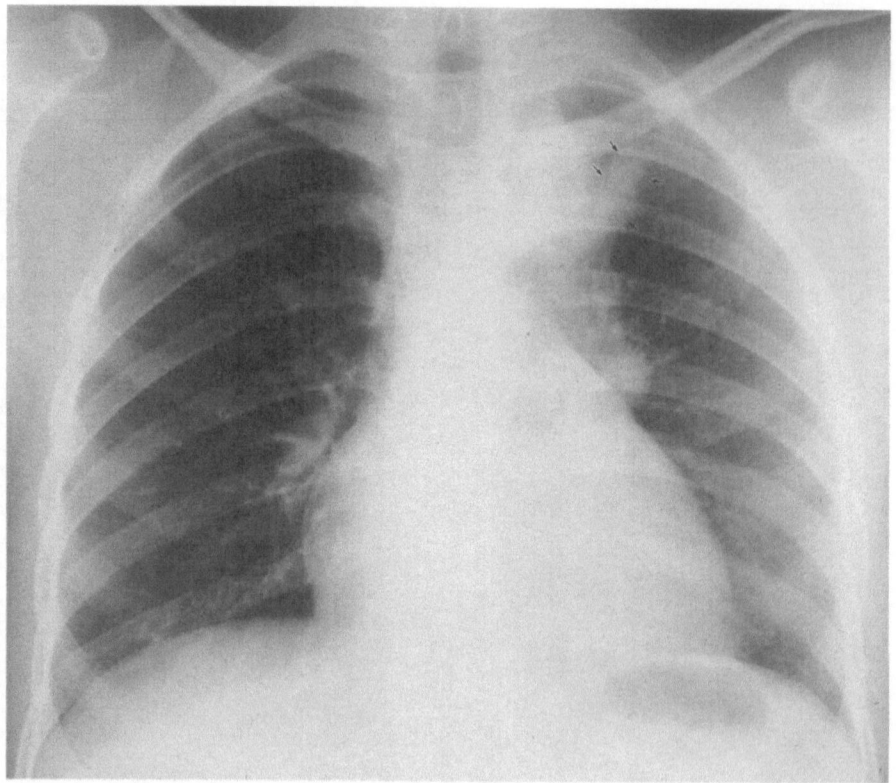

Fig. 3.2. CXR; primary TB with prominent paratracheal adenopathy, a full L hilar region and a parenchymal focus in the LUL (arrows). L rather than R paratracheal adenopathy is less common in primary TB.

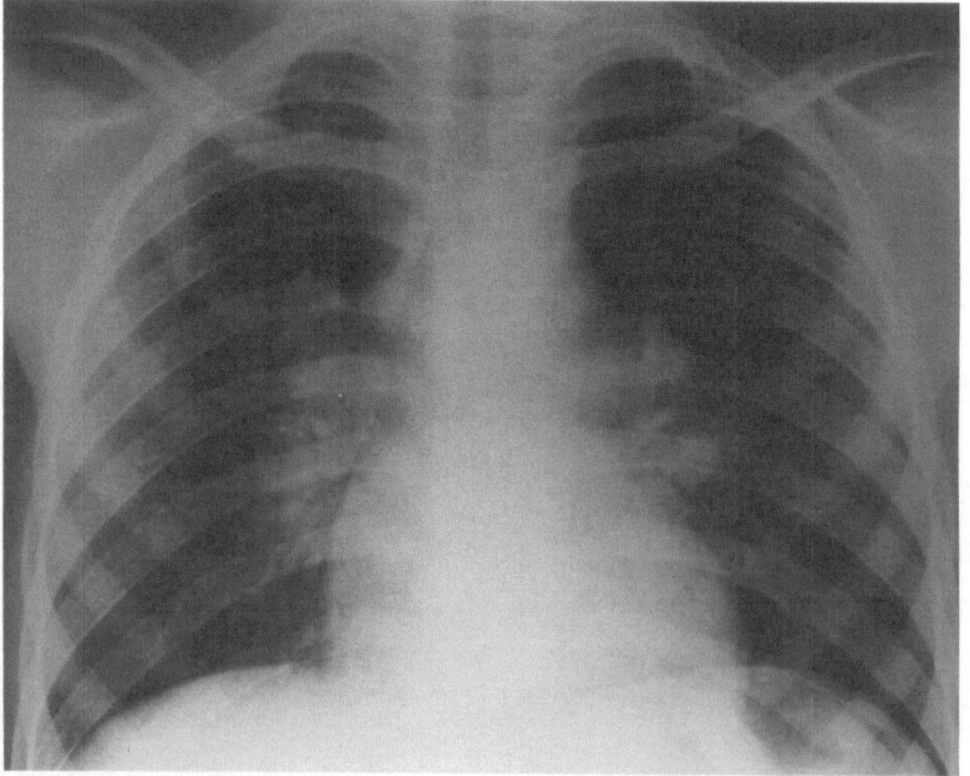

Fig. 3.3. CXR; primary TB with marked bilateral hilar adenopathy.

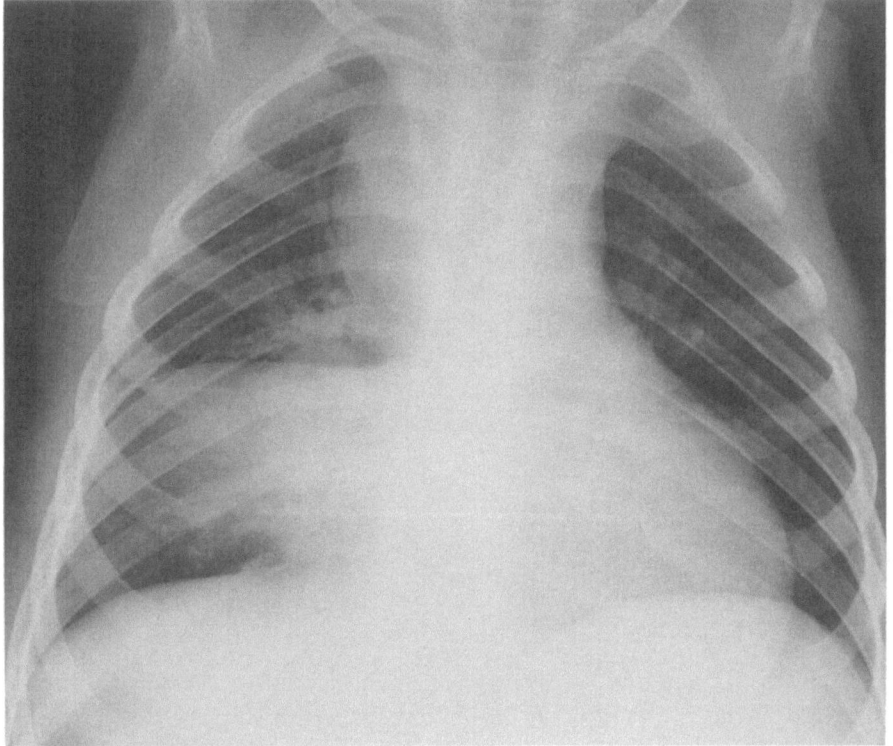

a

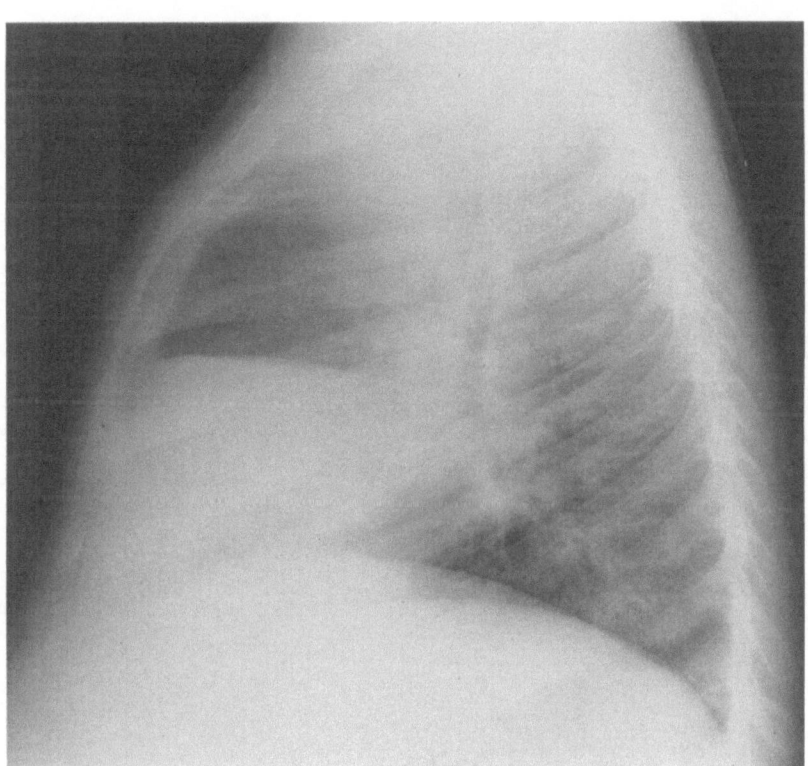

b

Fig. 3.4a, b. CXR AP and lateral; a characteristic appearance of TB with R paratracheal and R hilar adenopathy and opacification of the RML.

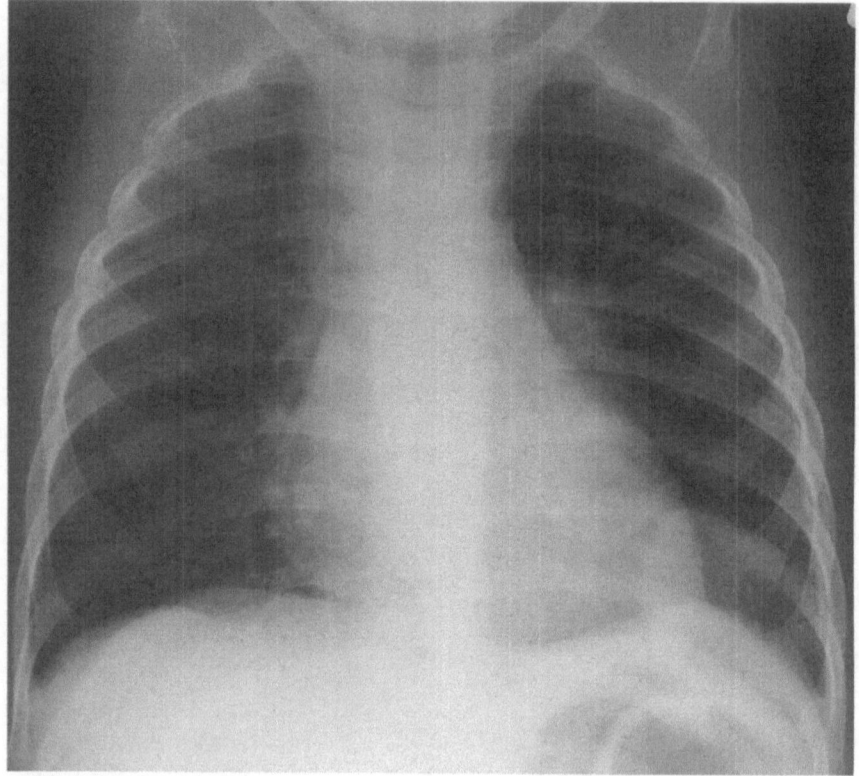

a

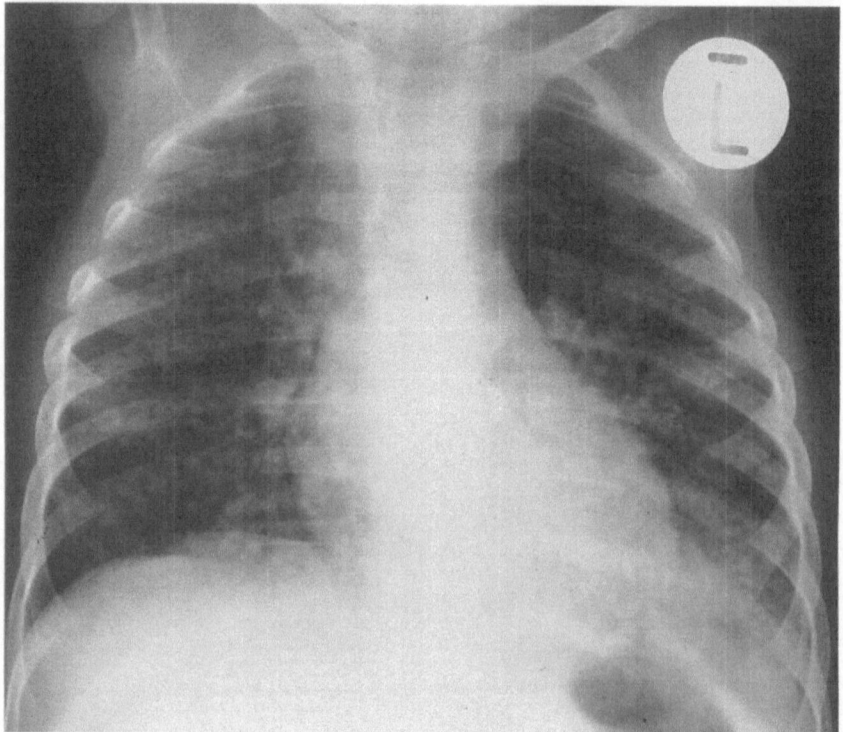

b

Fig. 3.5a, b. CXRs; **a** on presentation the child had a round focus of opacification in the LLL and was treated for bacterial pneumonia. The R paratracheal adenopathy was not initially appreciated (note the trachea central in the superior mediastinal opacification). **b** One week later a wide-spread reticular nodular pattern developed in keeping with acute hematogenous dissemination of TB.

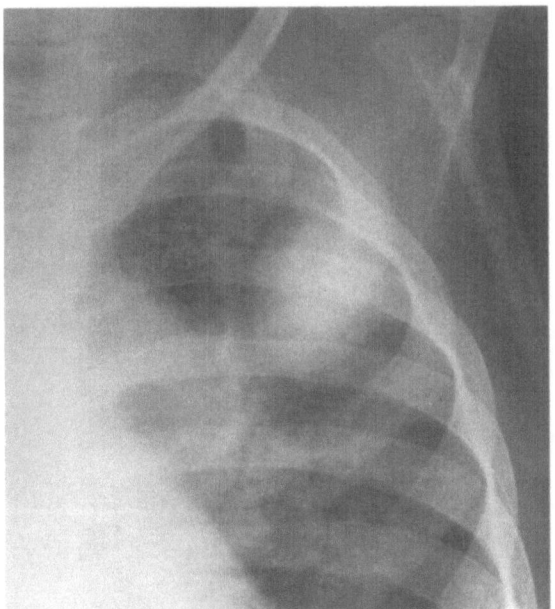

Fig. 3.6. CXR; Ghon focus in the LUL with L hilar adenopathy constituting a primary or Rankes complex.

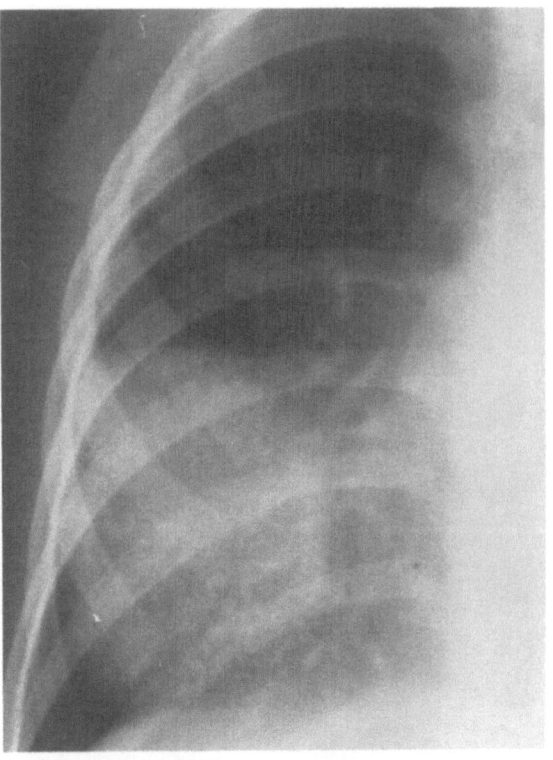

Fig. 3.8. CXR; RML is filled by a mass with calcific speckling typical of TB.

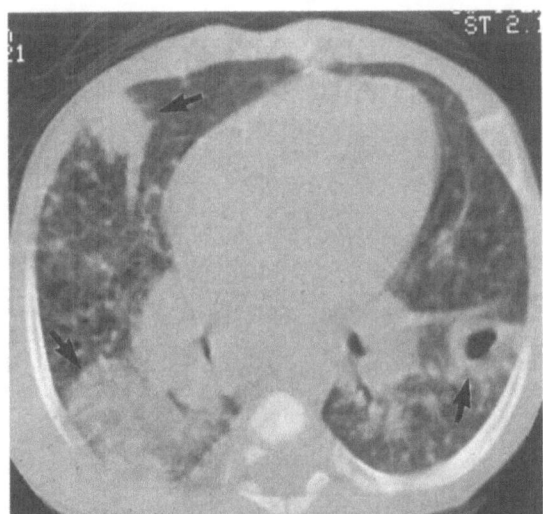

Fig. 3.7. CT; three foci of parenchymal opacification are noted (arrows) with bilateral hilar adenopathy. The R main bronchus is compromised and the RLL opacification may be a segmental lesion of lymphobronchial origin whilst the other two foci could be multifocal primary lesions. Note the L sided focus is cavitated (this was not apparent on CXR) and the wide-spread small nodules which are in keeping with acute disseminated TB.

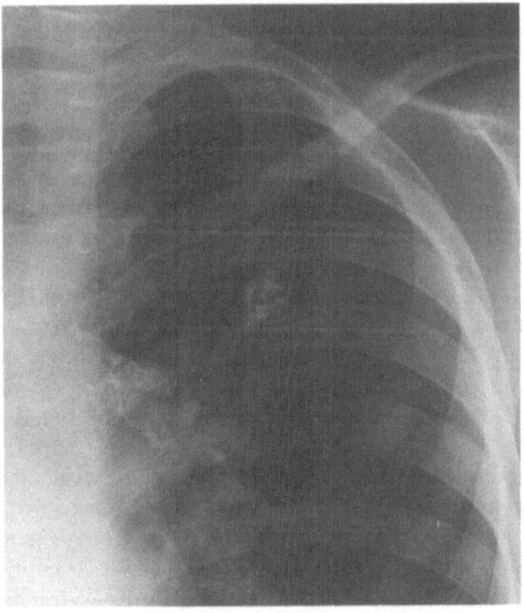

Fig. 3.9. CXR; calcified primary focus in the LUL and calcified lymph nodes result from a healed primary complex.

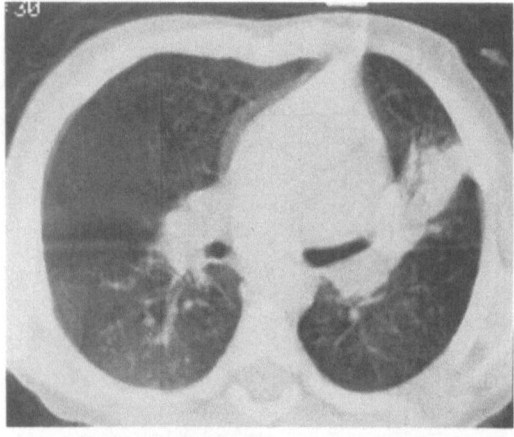

a

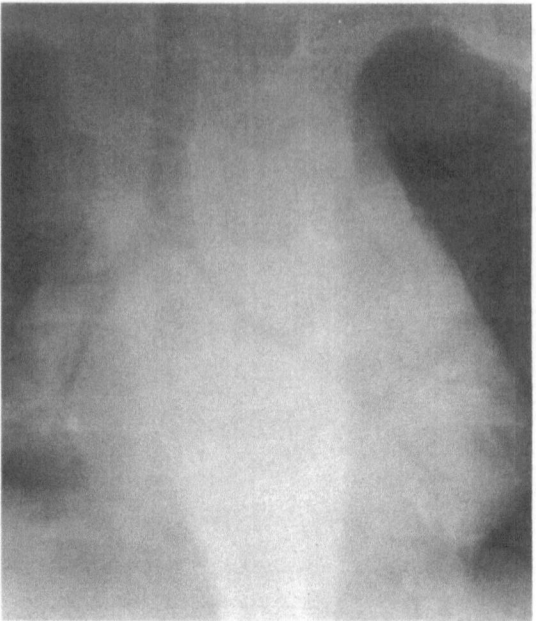

Fig. 3.11. High kV filtered X-ray; the L main bronchus is narrowed and stretched by a nodal mass with subcarinal component.

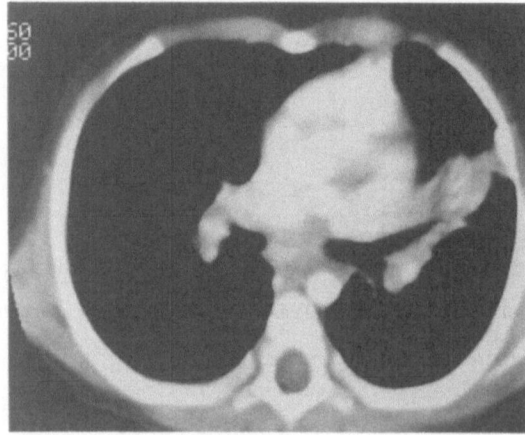

b

Fig. 3.10. a CT, b IV contrast-enhanced CT; L lingula opacification with no demonstrated adenopathy. The case did not respond to antibiotics but cleared on anti-TB medication. A clinical diagnosis of TB was felt to be likely.

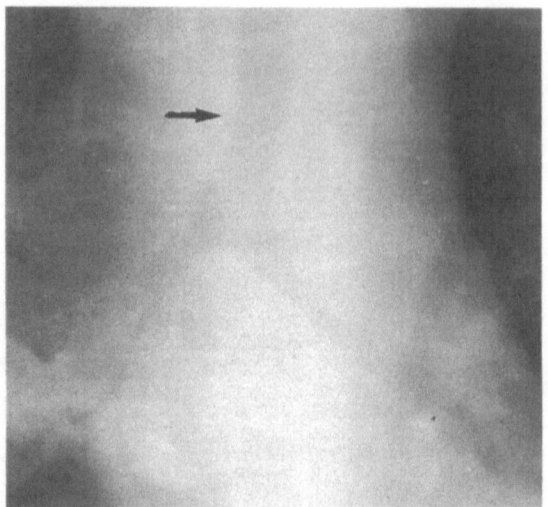

Fig. 3.12. High kV filtered X-ray; nodal impression on the trachea (arrow). Marked narrowing of the R bronchus intermedius and some compression of the L main bronchus.

On CXR, adenopathy is usually detected in the frontal projection and hilar adenopathy confirmed by the lateral projection. The detection of hilar node enlargement is not always easy. In general the adenopathy tends to be asymmetrical and often unilateral. The predominance of right hilar and right paratracheal adenopathy reflects the drainage of the right lung and the lower half of the left lung via this group of nodes.

Nodes may be sharply defined and lobulated or can be ill-defined with vague borders. Superior mediastinal widening in a child may be difficult to evaluate but in the subclavicular region a normal left-sided aortic arch should place the trachea to the right of the mediastinal opacificaton. A central trachea should raise suspicion of right paratracheal adenopathy (Fig. 3.5a). Displacement of the tracheobronchial tree is common with splaying of the carina by subcarinal adenopathy. This is well demonstrated by filtered high-kV radiographs (Figs 3.11, 3.12). Calcification is characteristic of TB and occurs in diseased parenchyma and lymph nodes. It may be present on initial CXR but usually takes at least 3–6 months to become apparent. Adenopathy may persist for 2 years or longer, and even on adequate therapy may initially enlarge.

Intravenous contrast-enhanced dynamic CT studies are very sensitive for detection of hilar and mediastinal lymph adenopathy (Figs 3.13, 3.14, 3.15, 3.16). Lymph node enlargement has been defined as >5 mm in children >4 years and >7 mm in children >8 years[15]. The authors have usually found them to be in the region of 1.5 cm, often presenting in matted clusters. Intravenous contrast enhancement highlights vascular structures and TB nodes characteristically show rim enhancement. Hypodense central areas may occur which reflect underlying necrosis[16]. Calcification is detected far earlier by CT than by CXR (Fig. 3.17). CT is also a good modality for separating adenopathy from other mediastinal mass lesions and is useful for evaluating equivocal CXRs where confirmation or exclusion of adenopathy is important for diagnosis and treatment.

Ultrasound can also be used to visualize mediastinal adenopathy, but more especially paratracheal or anterior mediastinum nodes (Fig. 3.18). In malnourished children with little mediastinal fat and

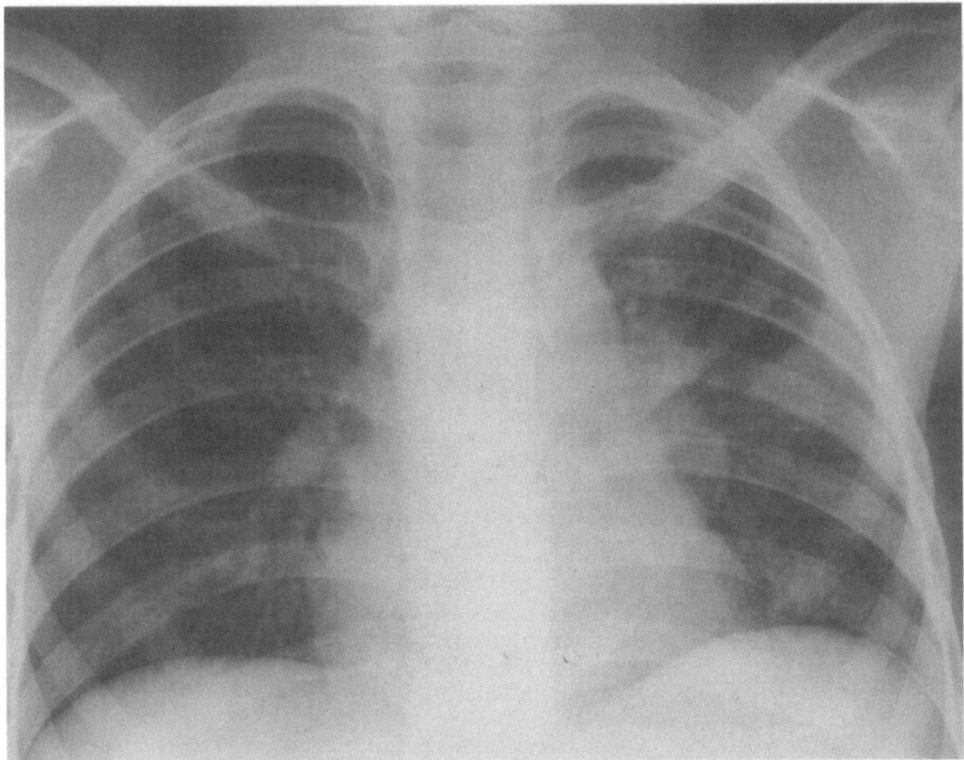

a

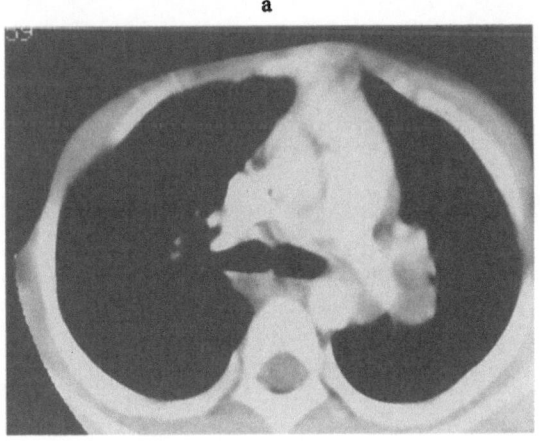

b

Fig. 3.13. a CXR, **b** IV contrast enhanced CT; L hilar opacity is confirmed on CT as rim-enhancing nodes.

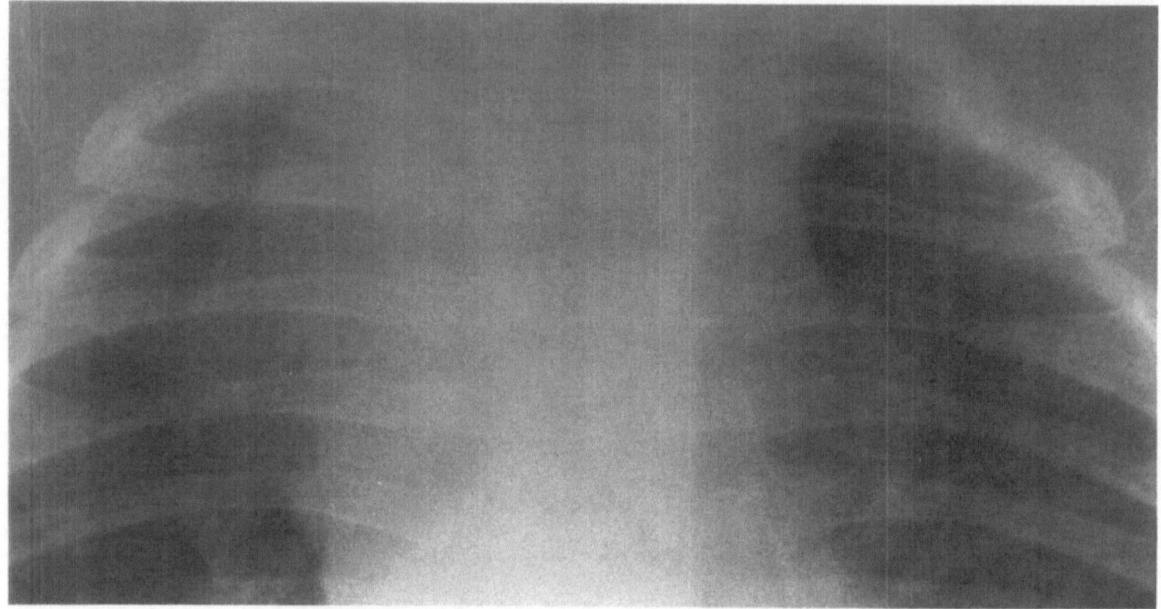

a

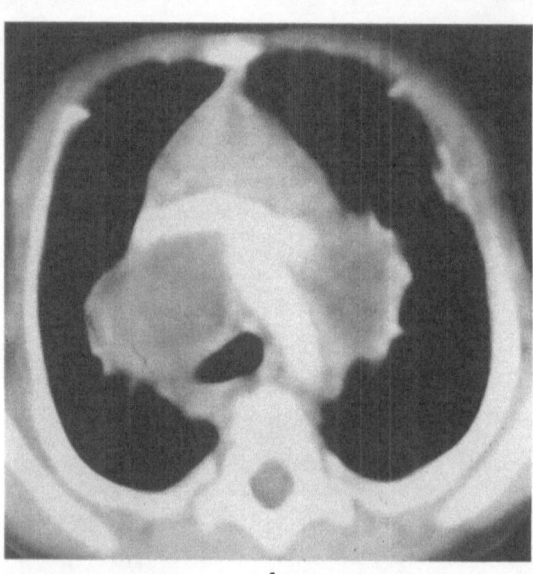

b

Fig. 3.14. a CXR, b IV contrast-enhanced CT; CT shows the widened superior mediastinum is clearly not thymus but large, rim-enhancing TB nodes.

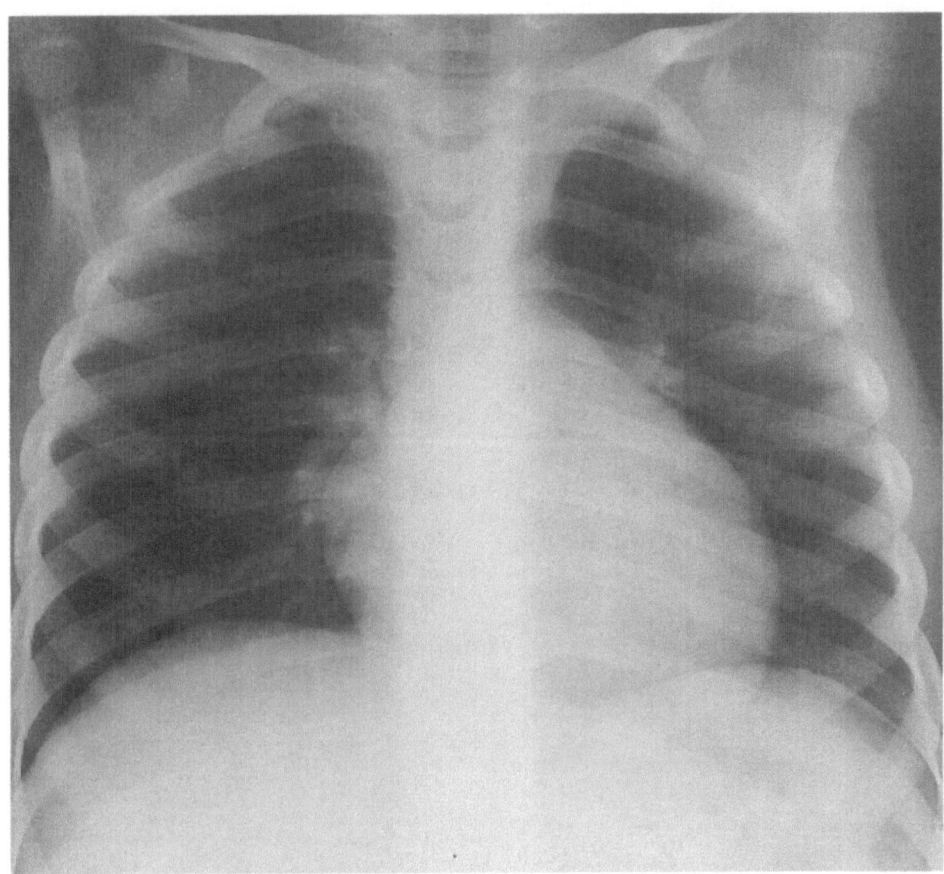

a

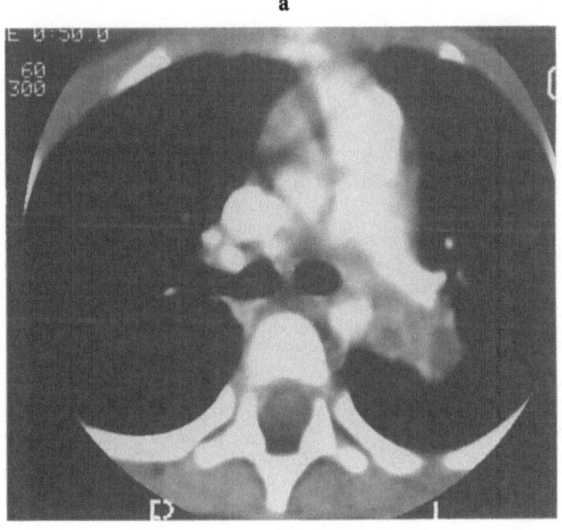

b

Fig. 3.15. a CXR, **b** IV contrast-enhanced CT; adenopathy not evident on CXR but CT clearly demonstrated rim-enhancing L hilar lymph nodes.

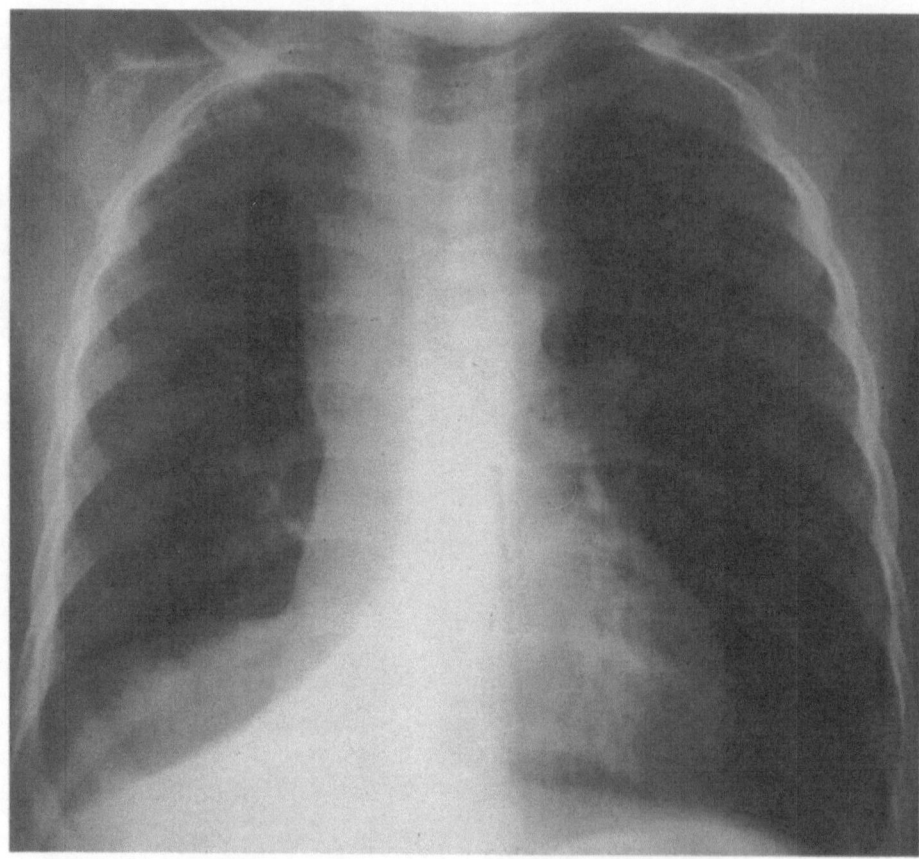

a

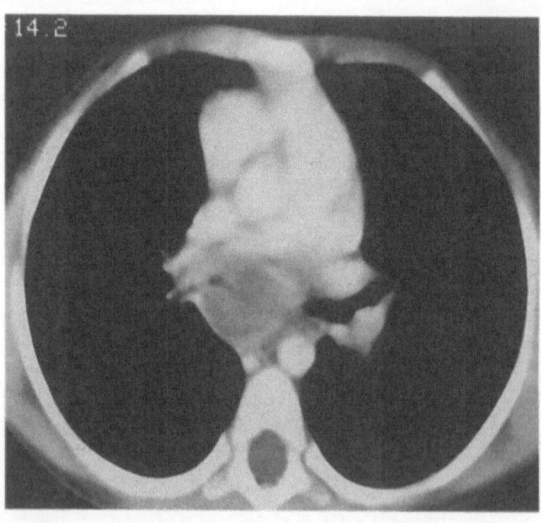

b

Fig. 3.16. a CXR, **b** IV contrast-enhanced CT; this child presented with a history of peanut ingestion and a foreign body obstruction of the R bronchus intermedius was suspected. CT demonstrates a large rim enhancing sub-carinal lymph node compressing the R bronchus intermedius.

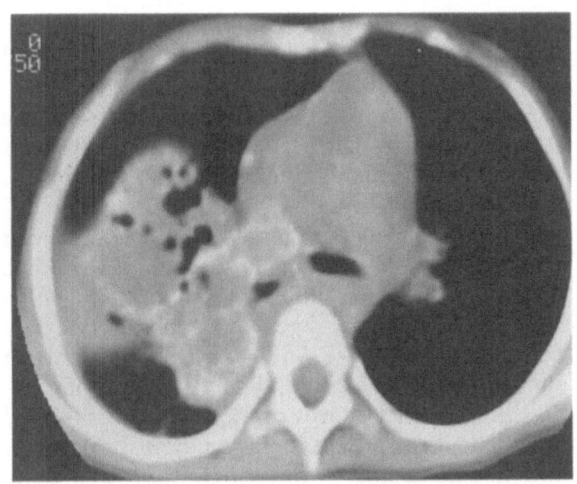

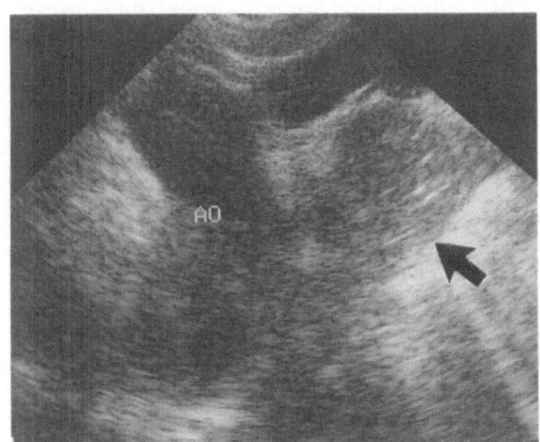

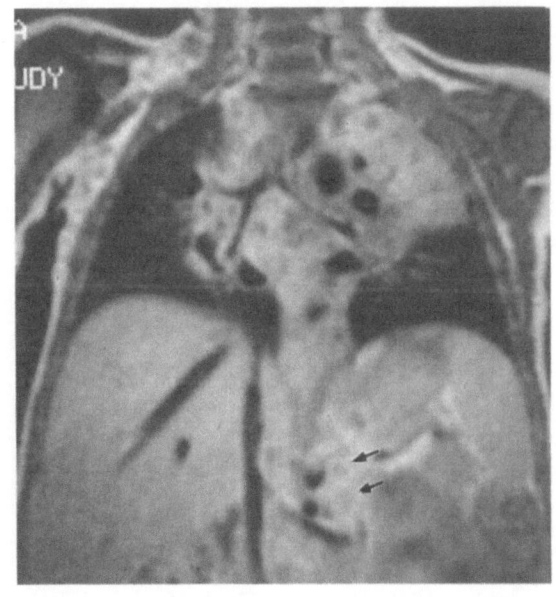

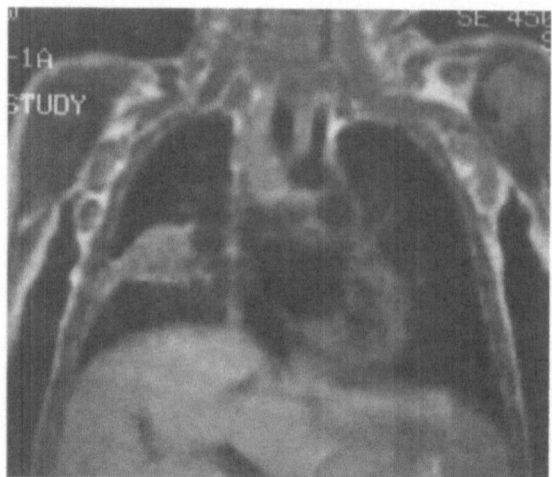

Fig. 3.20. Coronal IV gadolinium-enhanced T1 MR; segmental RML lesion and R paratracheal adenopathy is typical of TB.

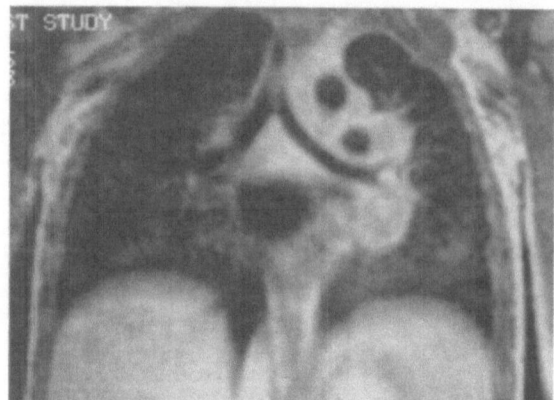

Fig. 3.21. Coronal IV gadolinium-enhanced T1 MR; rim-enhancing nodal masses of the L hilar area are well shown.

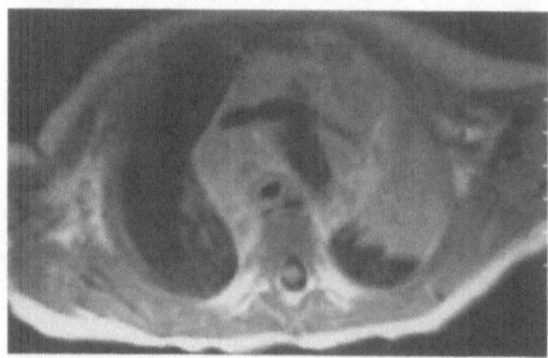

Fig. 3.22. Axial T1 MR; soft tissue of superior mediastinal adenopathy clearly distinguished from the aortic and subclavian veins. Consolidated LUL is present.

detection of calcification is poor, MR is a powerful modality for evaluation of mediastinal masses and only cost and availability restrict its use.

Adenopathy must be differentiated from the thymus, retrosternal thyroid, developmental cysts and solid mediastinal tumors, including neurogenic tumors, germ cell tumors and thymomas. The differential diagnosis of enlarged lymph nodes must also include lymphoma, especially Hodgkin's disease in the older child. These nodes tend to be large, lobulated, homogeneous, do not typically peripherally enhance with intravenous contrast studies and involve predominantly the anterior mediastinum. Other causes of metastatic adenopathy include leukemia, nephroblastoma, neuroblastoma and hepatoblastoma. Infectious entities include histoplasmosis, which may also calcify, other fungal infections and viral infections. HIV infection may present with adenopathy, and excluding TB is a diagnostic dilemma which imaging alone cannot resolve; similar difficulties occur in lymphoproliferative syndromes associated with immunotherapy, particularly in transplant patients. Histiocytosis may also have adenopathy as may sarcoidosis which is exceedingly rare in young children.

Progressive Primary/Lymphobronchial Disease

Lymphobronchial disease develops subsequent to the primary complex with parenchymal pathology occurring secondarily to lymph node involvement of the tracheo-bronchial tree. The anatomic proximity of the lymph node chains to the airways accounts for the high frequency of this complication. Adenopathy may partially or completely obstruct a bronchus or even the trachea (Figs 3.23, 3.24, 3.25). A wide spectrum of parenchymal abnormalities results from this pathology. These abnormalities include segmental or lobar consolidation, often with loss of volume (Figs 3.16, 3.23), but occasionally with "ball valve" hyperinflation (Fig. 3.26). Obstructed lobes also can develop secondary infection, which often precipitates presentation to hospital and may obscure the underlying TB infection. A node may also rupture into a bronchus discharging caseous material into the airways. This can result in bronchogenic spread down a single bronchus, giving a segmental lesion, or cause a wide-spread TB bronchopneumonia (Fig. 3.27). The differing reported incidence of segmental lesions (areas of consolidation with or without some degree of collapse) demonstrates the difficulties associated with "pattern" descriptions of primary TB.

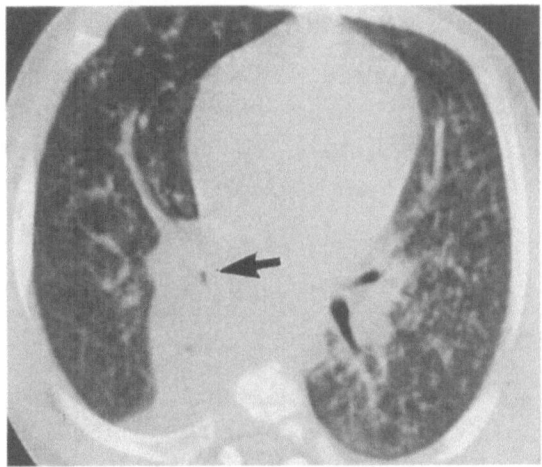

Fig. 3.23. CT; extreme nodal compression of the R lower lobe bronchus (arrow) with segmental consolidation and increased volume of the remaining RLL.

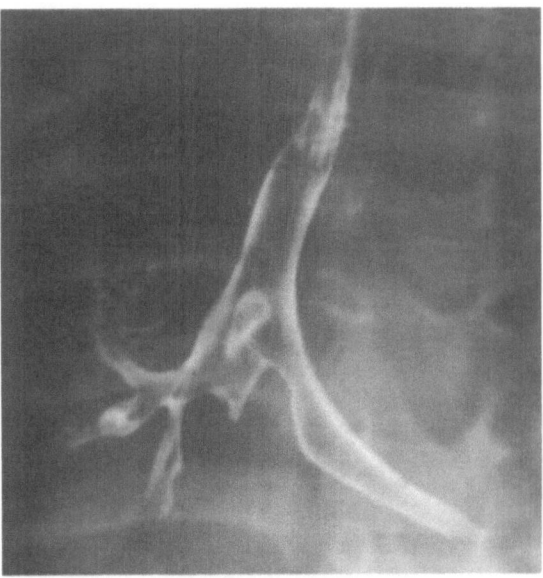

Fig. 3.25. Bronchogram; subcarinal nodal impression.

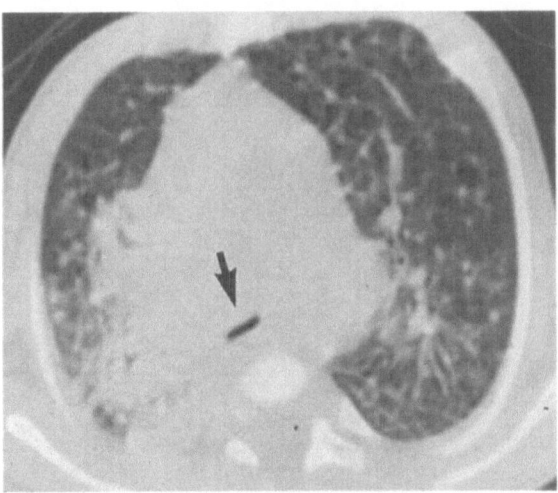

Fig. 3.24. CT; marked nodal compression of the trachea (arrow). RUL consolidation is present.

Segmental lesions are more common on the right, but their overall incidence varies from 28%[13] to 29%[10] and 56%[9] to 83%[17]. In the differential diagnosis must be included inhaled foreign bodies and other infections.

Although the incidence of cavitation reported by CXR is low, varying from 5%[15] to 14%[5] and 16%[14], the use of CT has shown cavitation or localized areas of breakdown to be far more common than seen on routine CXR even with retrospective insight. It is an indicator of disease activity and was seen frequently when CT was used in our selected problem-solving situations. CT has also been used to follow-up the progress of these lesions after treatment[18]. Pneumatoceles or cysts may occur in the parenchyma (Fig. 3.28); these more commonly occur in staphylococcal pneumonia, but in these cases the child is acutely ill. Both parenchymal lesions and adenopathy are slow to resolve, taking 6 months to 2 years to clear[9,12]. Parenchymal lesions tend to precede the resolution of adenopathy but residual calcific lung and nodal foci may remain indefinitely (Fig. 3.9).

A brief mention of bronchoscopy as a method of visualizing tuberculous lesions completes this survey. The examination is indicated in bronchial infection to clear a site of obstruction or to ensure that no foreign body is present. Miller has described four stages in the appearance and development of these lesions[19].

1. Local bulging of the bronchial wall with circumferential redness and swelling.

2. Local bulging with protruding yellow areas.

3. Blockage of the lumen by granulation tissue and caseous material.

4. An erosion through which caseous material may be seeping.

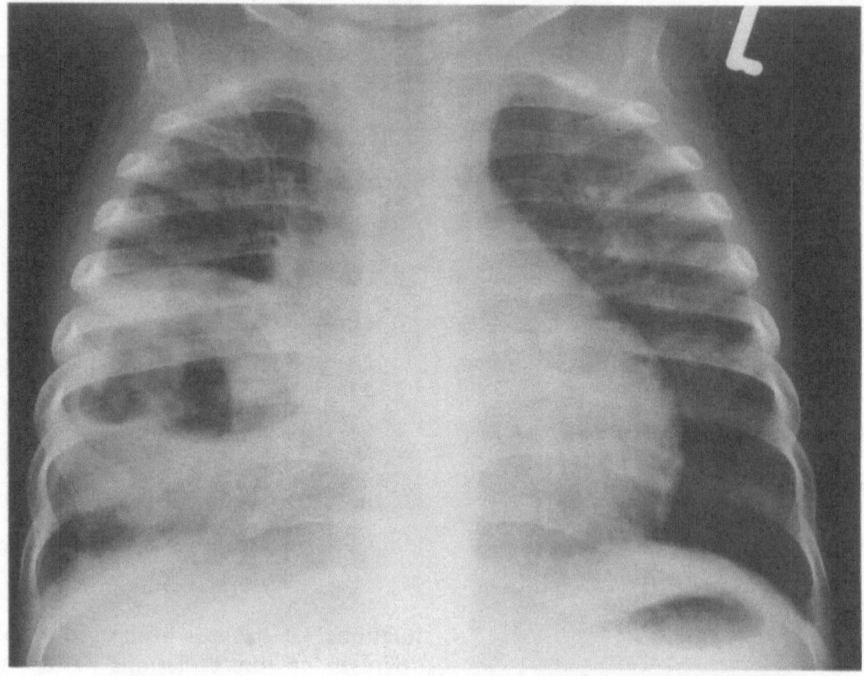

a

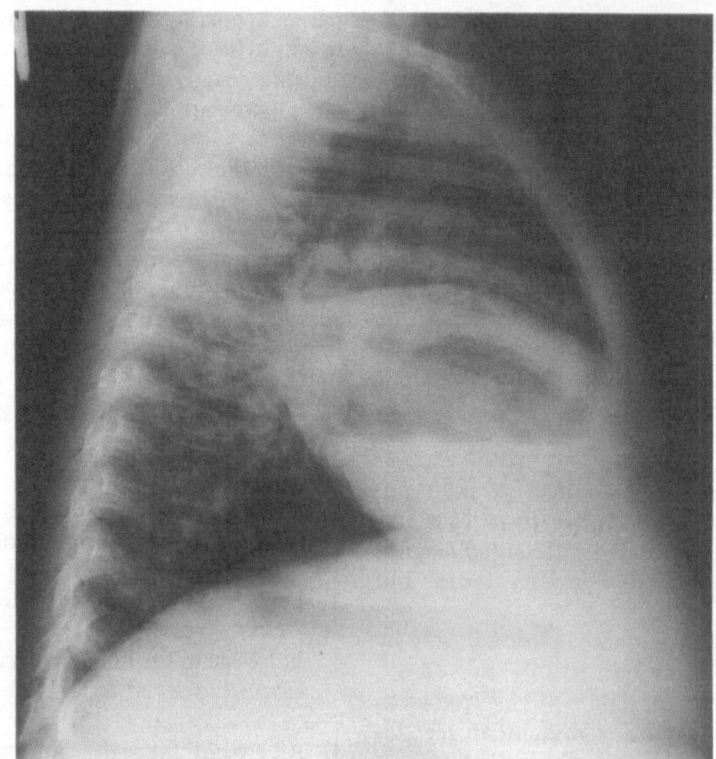

b

Fig. 3.26a, b. CXR; the consolidated RML has a large cavity and hyperinflated with bulging convex fissures. R paratracheal adenopathy indents the trachea.

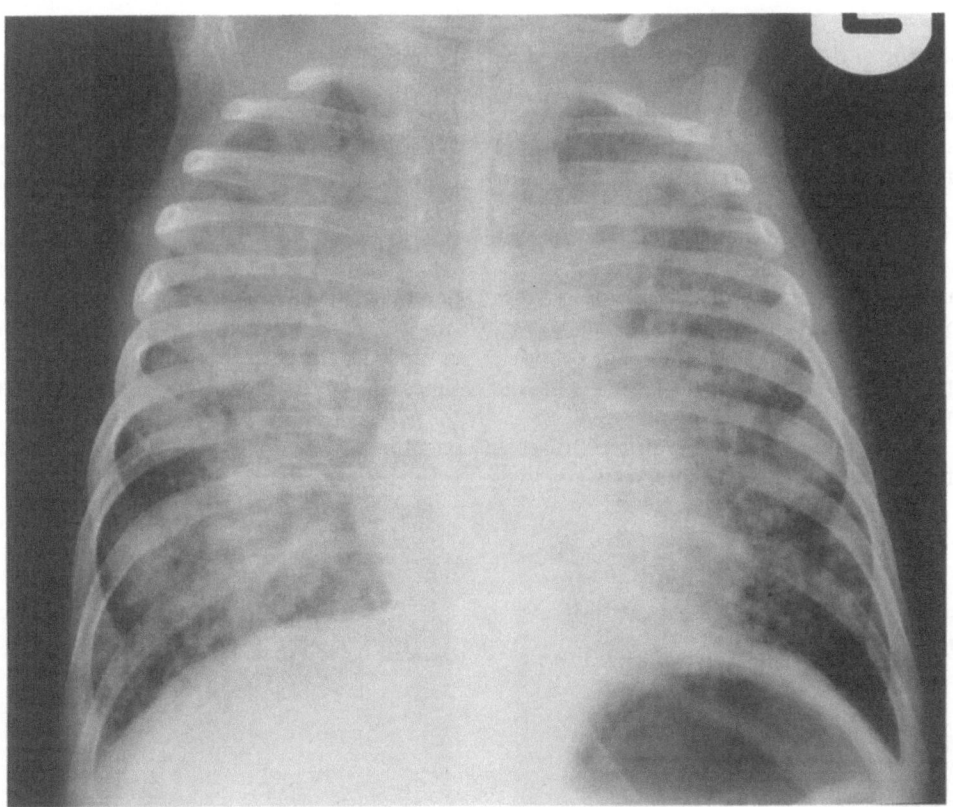

Fig. 3.27. CXR; bilateral TB bronchopneumonia.

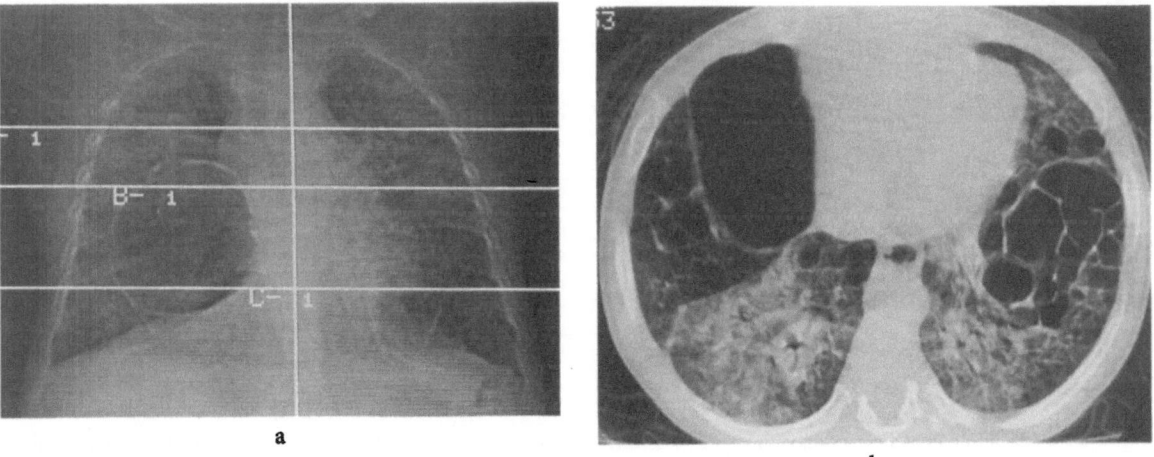

Fig. 3.28. a Digital CT surview CXR, **b** CT; an enlarging parenchymal cyst of the RML that required surgical decompression. CT revealed far more widely spread cystic changes in both lungs than CXR suggested.

Late Parenchymal Disease

Lung lobes (or entire lung) may be destroyed by progressive TB infection, associated secondary infection or adenopathy causing bronchus or vascular compression. Some of these patients will require surgical management and CT helps to define the anatomic extent of diseased lung, which is of importance if resection is contemplated, and to ensure the normality of remaining lung (Fig. 3.29).

Bronchiectasis is a serious delayed complication. The radiological appearance of bronchiectasis is irreversible airway dilatation with a cystic or cylindrical pattern. It is clinically supported by chronic sputum production and the development of finger clubbing. This is relevant as symptomatic disease with confirmed radiologic bronchiectasis requires

evaluation for surgery, whilst an asymptomatic patient with dilated airways which clear and drain themselves may not. The insult and damage to the bronchi may occur during acute disease from bronchus obstruction or bronchial stenosis resulting from fibrosis, which occurs with healing of granulomatous lesions. CXR shows persistent opacification and atelectasis with dilated and cystic airways. Currently there is a lack of a suitable contrast medium for bronchography in children so that HRCT studies with collimated thin slices are used to demonstrate bronchiectasis and its anatomic location[20,21]. A narrow window width has to be selected to accentuate the abnormalities[21], and fast scan times are advantageous as motion artefacts disturb the width of pulmonary vessels and blur the edges of small bronchial walls. CT interpretation needs considerable experience. Dilated bronchi that run hori-

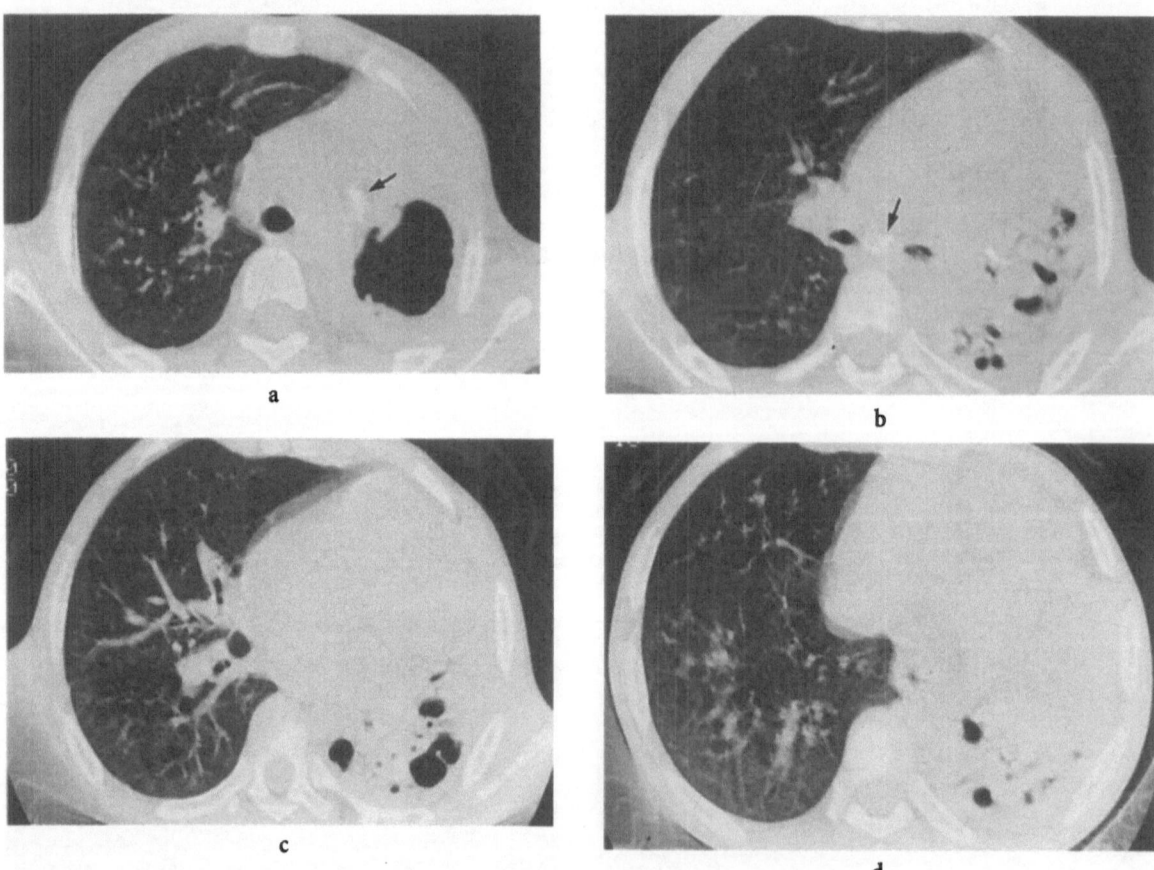

Fig. 3.29 a–d. CT; L lung destruction with volume loss cavitation and consolidation. Calcification of LUL and subcarinal regions are present (arrows). The R lung shows no gross pathology and the patient has done well following L pneumonectomy.

zontally appear as "tram lines" (Fig. 3.30), whilst those orientated vertically appear as thick-walled lucencies, and when adjacent to pulmonary arteries have a "signet ring" appearance[21] (Fig. 3.31). In atelectasis the circular or elongated bronchi are bunched together. Mucoid impaction in bronchi and thin-walled cystic bronchi may present difficulties in interpretation, but identification is assisted by recognition of peripherally situated airways that are larger than adjacent pulmonary arteries.

Reactivation or reinfection of an immune-competent host gives rise to the "adult" type of TB with a cavitating, fibrotic disease, predominantly affecting the apices without regional lymphadenopathy (Fig. 3.32). We have not seen this appearance in prepubertal children.

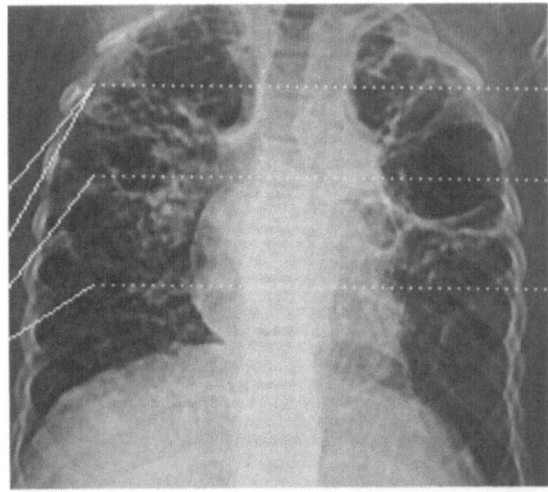

a

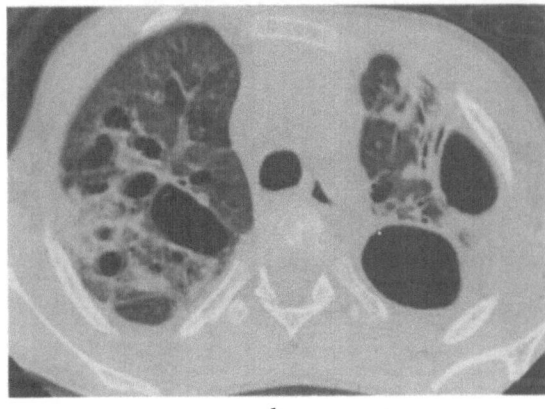

b

Fig. 3.32. a Digital CT surview CXR, **b** HRCT; 12-year-old sputum positive for TB with fibrotic cavitating apices and no evidence of adenopathy. The appearance of "adult" TB.

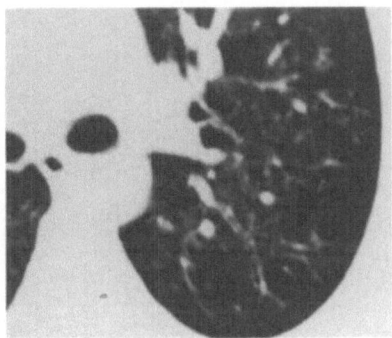

Fig. 3.30. HRCT; post-TB bronchiectasis LLL. Airways not narrowing down in the periphery form "tram lines" (arrow).

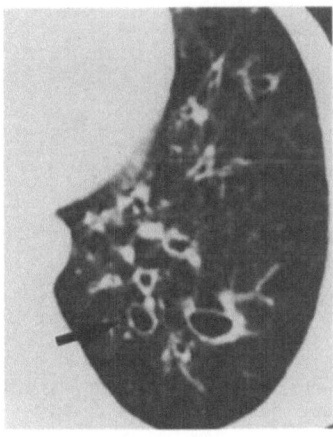

Fig. 3.31. HRCT; post-TB bronchiectasis LLL. Note the disproportion in size between airway and associated pulmonary artery (arrow), the "signet ring" sign.

Acute Disseminated Disease

A liquified caseating focus, usually nodal, rupturing into a blood vessel will precipitate a massive bacillemia. The resultant disseminated disease is known as "miliary" TB. The preferable term is "acute disseminated disease", as "miliary" is used with reference to the CXR[22]. The word miliary has its origin in the small, approximately 2-mm, round, whitish millet seeds to which early pathologists likened the granulomas found at autopsy. The CXR appearances are variable and the spectrum varies from a normal CXR, through an interstitial-nodular pattern to the common diffuse confluent patchy irregular nodular pattern or "snowstorm" appearance[23]. The traditional or classical "miliary pattern" (a collection of tiny, discrete,

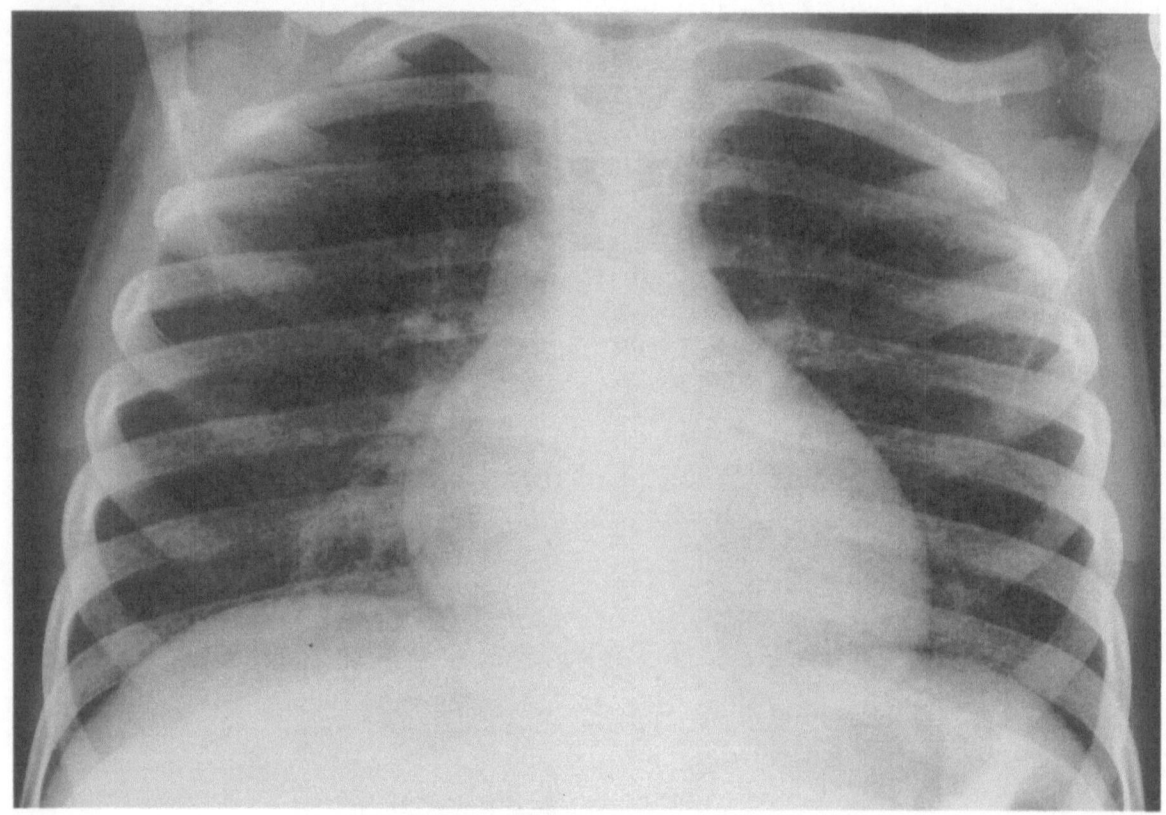

a

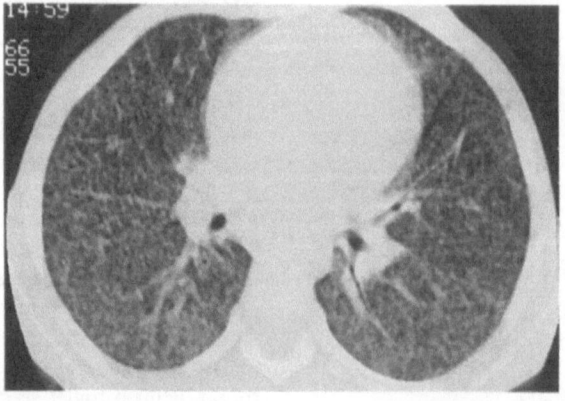

b

Fig. 3.33. a CXR; acute disseminated tuberculosis with fine reticular nodular lung pattern (miliary pattern) and **b** HRCT showing small, widespread nodules with a predominant pattern of interlobular septal and interstitial thickening.

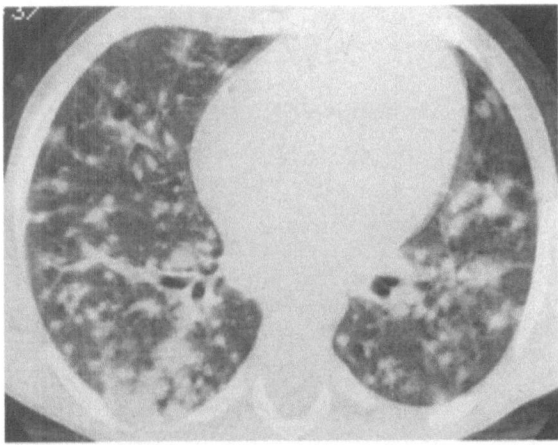

Fig. 3.34. HRCT; acute disseminated disease with larger nodules, a more sparse distribution and evidence of coalescing nodules in the RLL. Interlobular septal thickening is present.

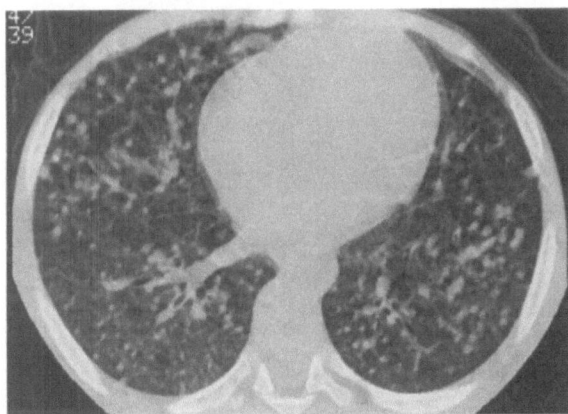

Fig. 3.35. HRCT; acute disseminated disease with nodules of two sizes suggesting two episodes of hematogenous dissemination.

pulmonary opacities that are generally uniform in size and measure 2 mm or less, as defined by the Fleishner Society[24]) is seldom seen in our young children. The authors' experience with HRCT in children with acute disseminated disease also shows great variation in appearance (Figs 3.33, 3.34, 3.35, 3.36). There are nodules of varying size and number, often with confluence and there is an interstitial component with interlobular septal thickening which may vary greatly in prominence[22]. The differentiation between diffuse hematogenous and diffuse bronchogenic spread may be difficult and

both methods of dissemination may be present at the same time, especially when cavitation is present (Fig. 3.37a, b). There is a significant increase of meningitis with acute hematogenous dissemination, (19%)[25], and mortality rate figures of the diffuse disease vary between 14%[25] and 56%[26]. Early diagnosis is an important factor in reducing this mortality rate[25].

Pleural Disease

A small juxta pleural focus is liable to release tuberculoprotein, which causes pleural inflammatory reaction and results in a clear protein-rich fluid and a painless pleural effusion, usually unilateral (Fig. 3.38). Effusions are considered more common in adolescents and adults[4,5] and the reported incidence in young children is between 4 to 6%[12] and 12%[10,13]. Interlobar effusions are isolated collections in the fissures from a localized reaction, or the end result of a larger resolving effusion.

A pleural empyema is not common, but it may occur. In primary progressive disease this results from either secondary infection or the rupture of a caseous node or necrotic lung into the pleural cavity (Fig. 3.39). Empyemas must be differentiated from other causes such as staphylococcal infection and it should be remembered that a cultured bacterial growth may be a secondary infection with TB the underlying primary infection (Ch 7, p. 109).

Ultrasound evaluates the pleural collections well (Fig. 3.40). CT has the advantage of evaluating lung and mediastinal structures hidden by the loculated fluid (Fig. 3.41) and localizes the effusion for efficient drainage. Complications of drainage procedures are also well imaged by CT (Figs 3.42, 3.43).

Pericardial Disease

The pericardium becomes involved secondarily to infection from contiguous mediastinal lymph nodes. In the Cape Town, South Africa community TB is a common cause of pericardial effusion[27], which may be large (Fig. 3.44). Evaluation by US is a simple procedure (Fig. 3.45) but CT is useful when ultrasonic access is limited by parenchymal or pleural pathology. CT also demonstrates well pericardial thickening and calcification (Fig. 3.46).

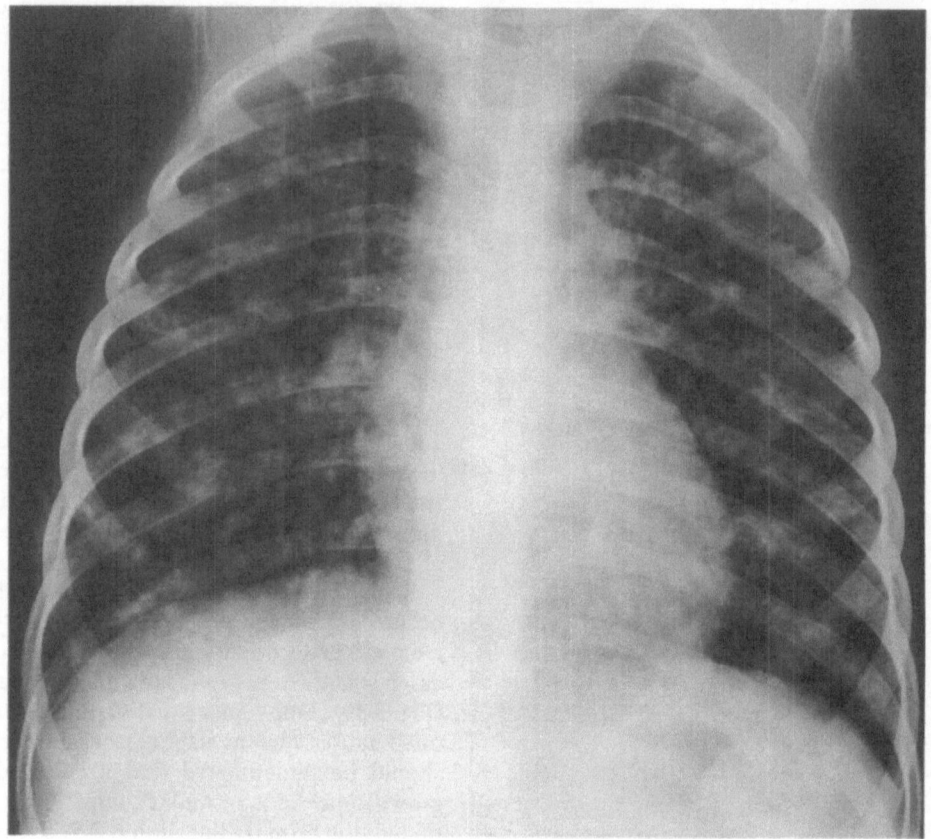

a

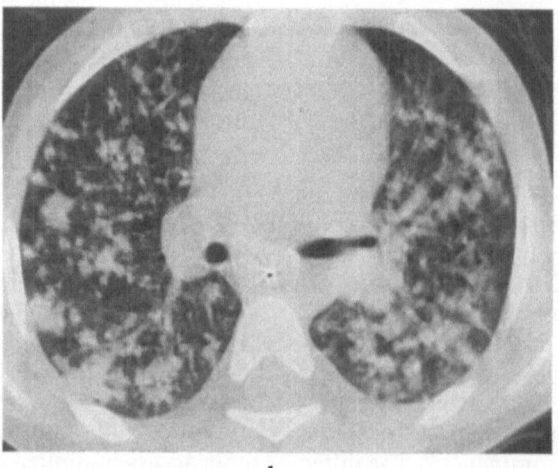

b

Fig. 3.36. a CXR, **b** HRCT; acute disseminated TB with a "snowstorm" interstitial nodular CXR pattern and HRCT demonstrating coalescence of nodules and interlobular septal thickening.

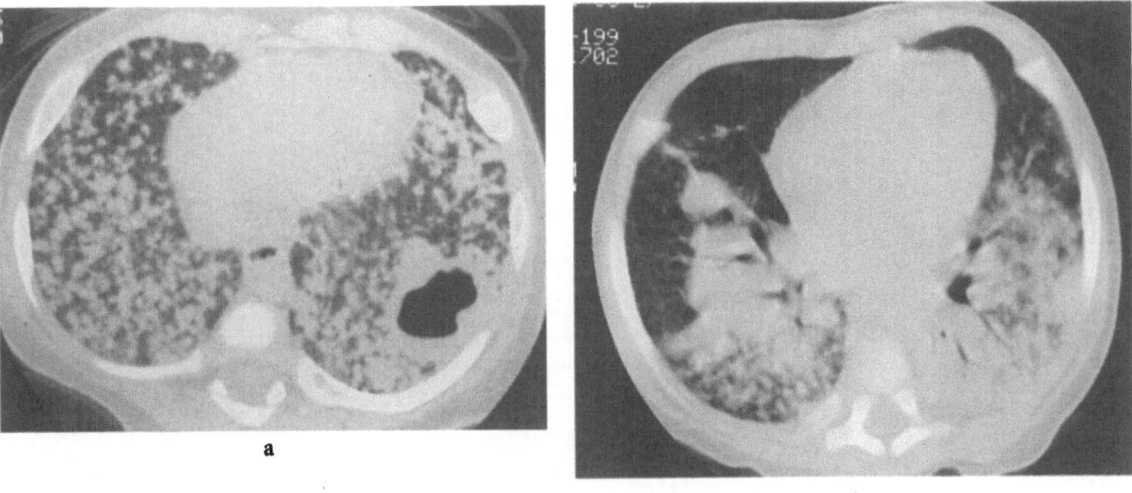

a

b

Fig. 3.37a, b. HRCT; these two patients demonstrate the difficulty in differentiating bronchogenic from hematogenous spread in acute disseminated TB. **a** had a uniform wide-spread nodular pattern suggestive of hematogenous spread, yet had a large pulmonary cavity and no overt extra-pulmonary TB whilst **b** had a confluent posterior basal opacification with nodular elements suggestive of bronchogenic spread, yet clinically the child presented with TB meningitis and hepatosplenomegaly.

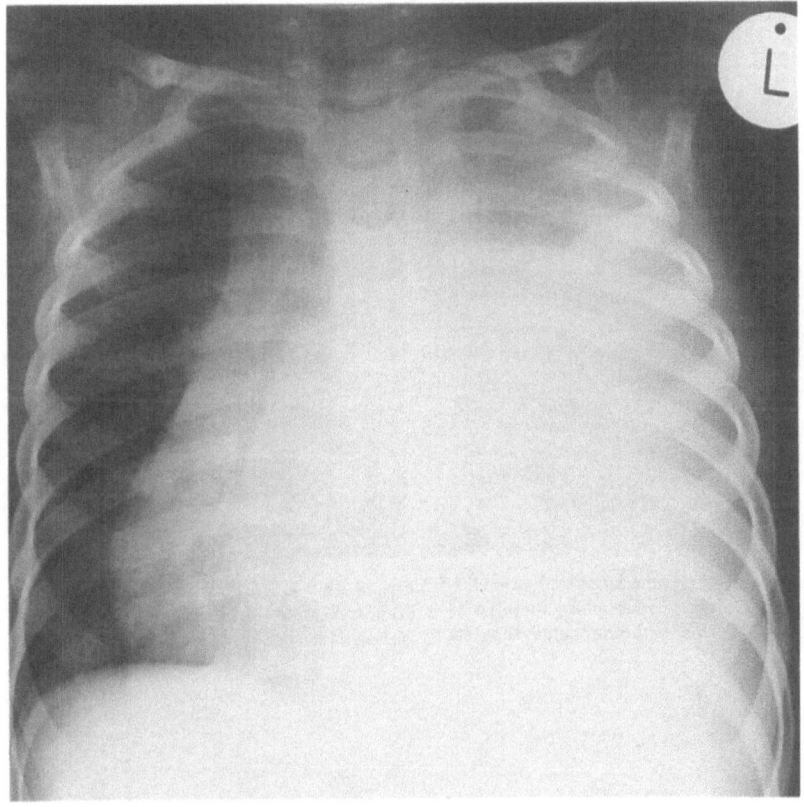

Fig. 3.38. CXR; a large L-sided TB pleural effusion displacing heart and mediastinum to the R.

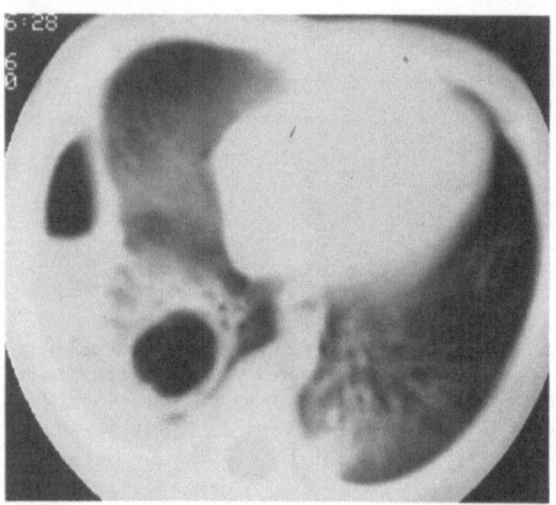

Fig. 3.39. CT; the cavities seen on CXR are clearly placed anatomically with both a pleural empyema and a parenchymal cavity.

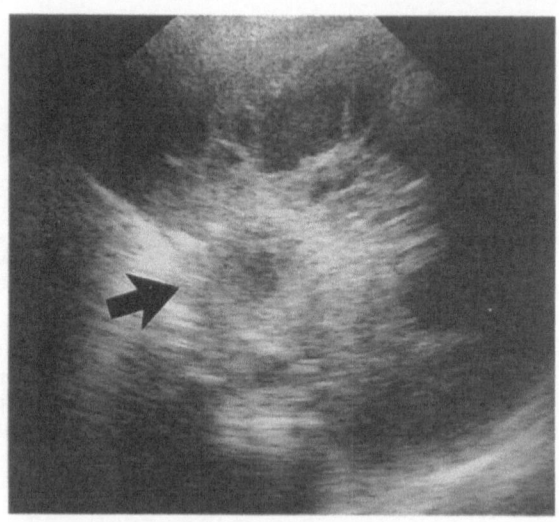

Fig. 3.40. US; imaging between the ribs easily demonstrates pleural fluid, the collapsed lung is seen (arrow). Placing of drains or biopsy is easily facilitated.

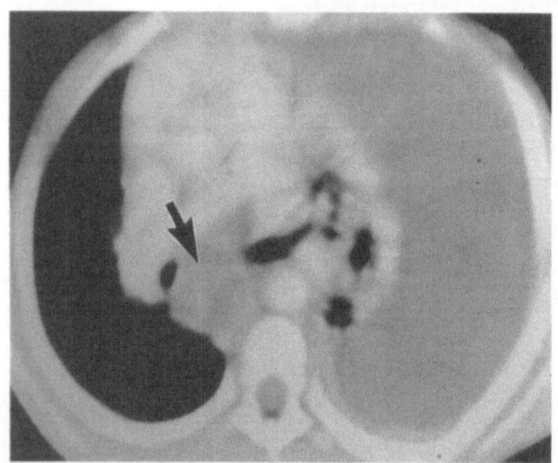

Fig. 3.41. IV contrast-enhanced CT; the large L pleural effusion obscured the collapsed L lung and adenopathy on plain X-ray. CT clearly demonstrates this pathology and suggests diagnosis of TB.

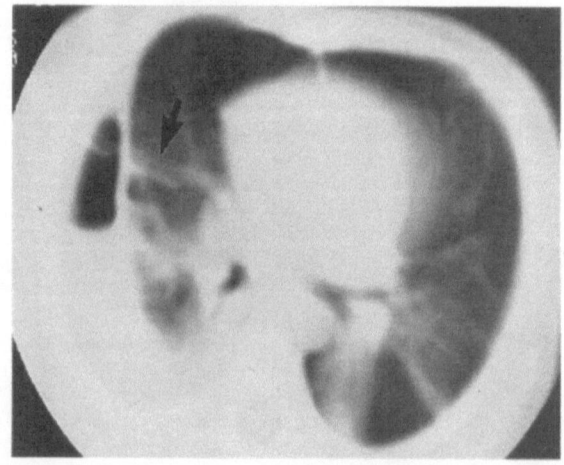

Fig. 3.42. CT; CT allows assessment of pleural drains and a drain traversing the pleural empyema and embedded in the lung is shown (arrow).

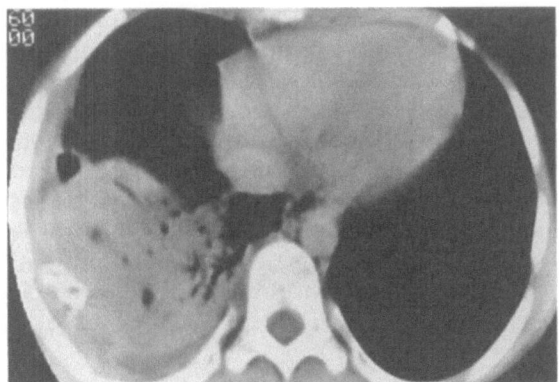

Fig. 3.43. CT; CT shows the pleural collection is drained and residual CXR opacification is parenchymal consolidation. The drains can be removed and not resited.

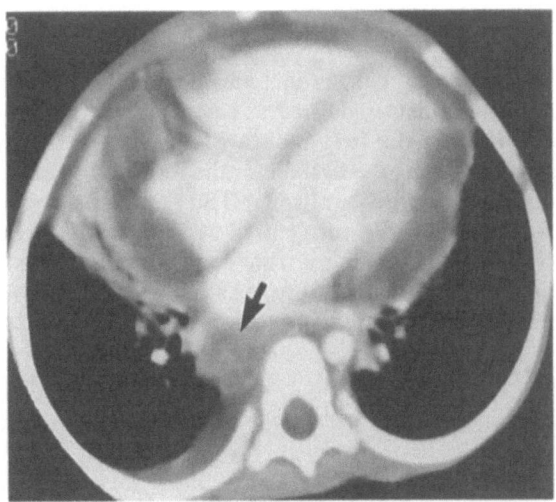

Fig. 3.44. IV contrast-enhanced CT; large TB pericardial effusion is well demonstrated. Segmental RML consolidation is present with a large TB lymph node clearly shown (arrow).

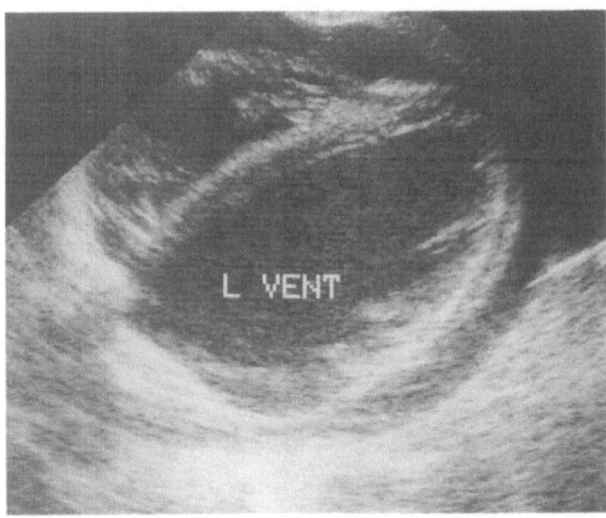

Fig. 3.45. US; US readily identifies pericardial fluid.

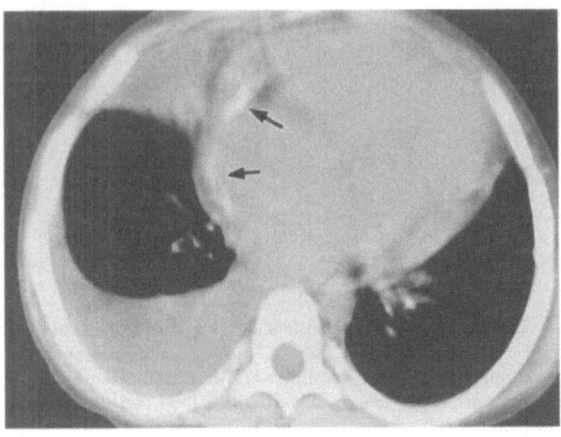

Fig. 3.46. CT; pericardial calcification is well depicted by CT (arrows). R pleural effusion and RML consolidation obscured the US access in this patient.

Neonatal Tuberculosis

Neonatal tuberculosis includes congenital TB and has been considered rare[28-31]. Neonatal by definition covers only the first month of life, but a recent series covering the first 3 months reported 38 cases of infants[31] with confirmed TB, 7 of which were considered to be congenital. It is difficult to be certain which cases are truly congenital, i.e., infection transmitted in utero, as they may have contracted the infection immediately after birth. The

Beitzke criteria[30] of a demonstrable primary in the neonatal liver with a positive tissue culture growth has been abandoned. It has been noted that infants born of infected mothers with tuberculous placentas do not usually develop neonatal disease[30]. More important is the recognition that neonatal cases may indicate previously unsuspected infection in mothers. The infants frequently have hepatosplenomegaly, and jaundice may also be present[31]. The imaging appearances are usually non-specific (Fig. 47a, b).

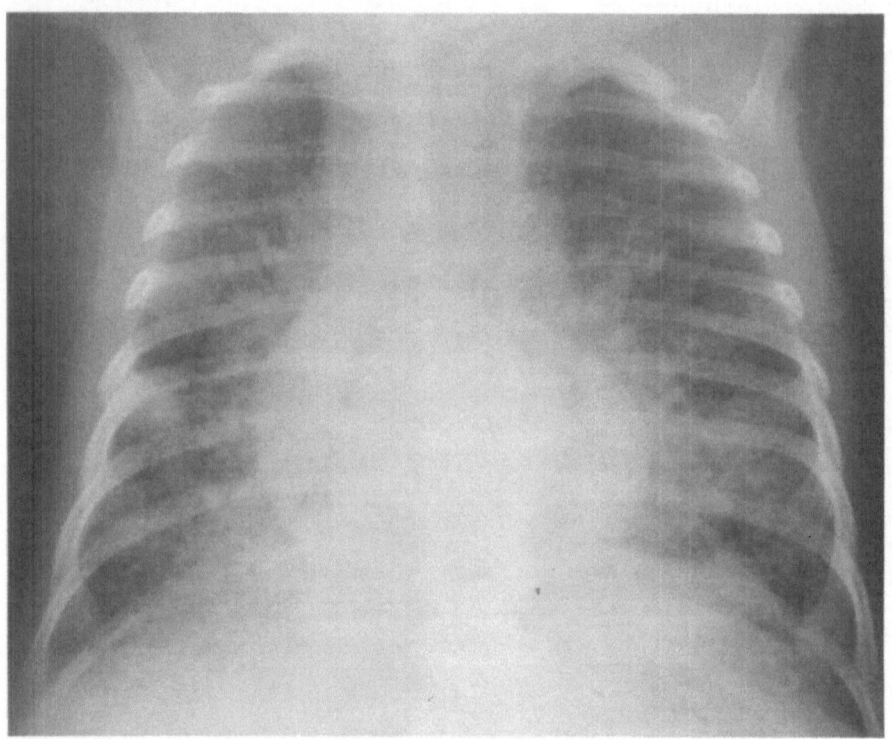

a

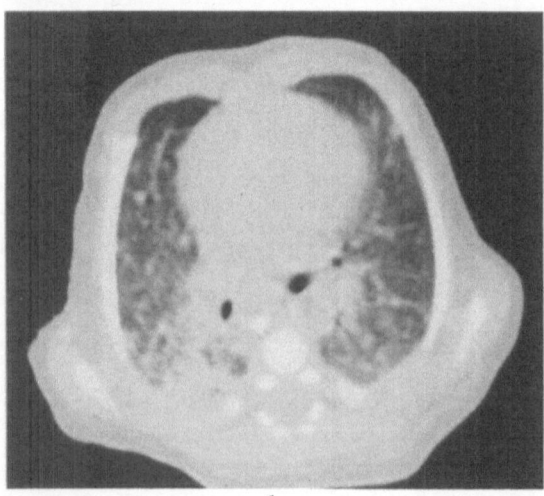

b

Fig. 3.47. a CXR, **b** CT; Neonatal TB, a neonate presented with respiratory distress at 2 weeks. Non-specific findings of a bronchopneumonia with parahilar and RLL infiltrate was found. The mother's CXR showed fibrotic upper lobe cavities typical of post-primary TB and bronchial washings in the child revealed innumerable acid-fast bacilli subsequently cultured for Mb TB.

Other Rare Manifestations

Tuberculous involvement of the larynx causes granulomatous mass lesions and is in the differential diagnosis of laryngeal tumors (Fig. 3.48). Mediastinal lymph nodes may rarely involve the phrenic nerve resulting in phrenic nerve palsy and an elevated diaphragm with inappropriate movement (best evaluated by direct screening when comparison of diaphragms is possible). Nodal involvement of the thoracic duct may result in chylothorax (Fig. 3.49). Necrosis and breakdown of matted mediastinal nodes may result in esophageal bronchial fistula formation which requires surgical management (Fig. 3.50a, b).

Resolution of Lesions

Lesions may take several months to clear and there may even be a paradoxical worsening of radiographic findings[12,32]. Parenchymal abnormalities should be evaluated every 2–3 months until cleared, but lymphadenopathy resolution may take considerably longer[32].

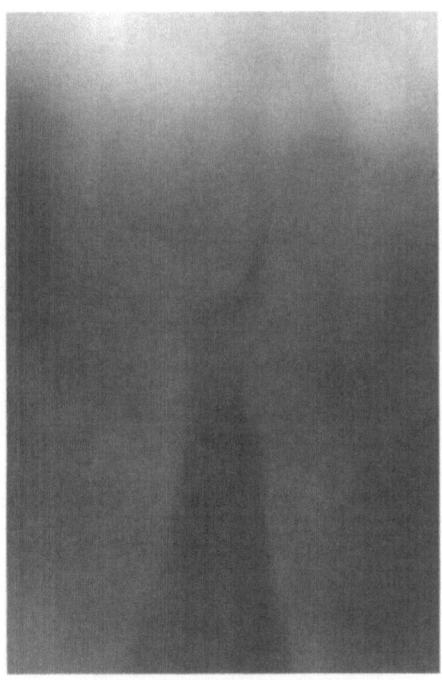

Fig. 3.48. Coronal linear tomograms; laryngeal tuberculosis presented in an adolescent with upper airway obstruction and granulomatous mass lesion in the larynx.

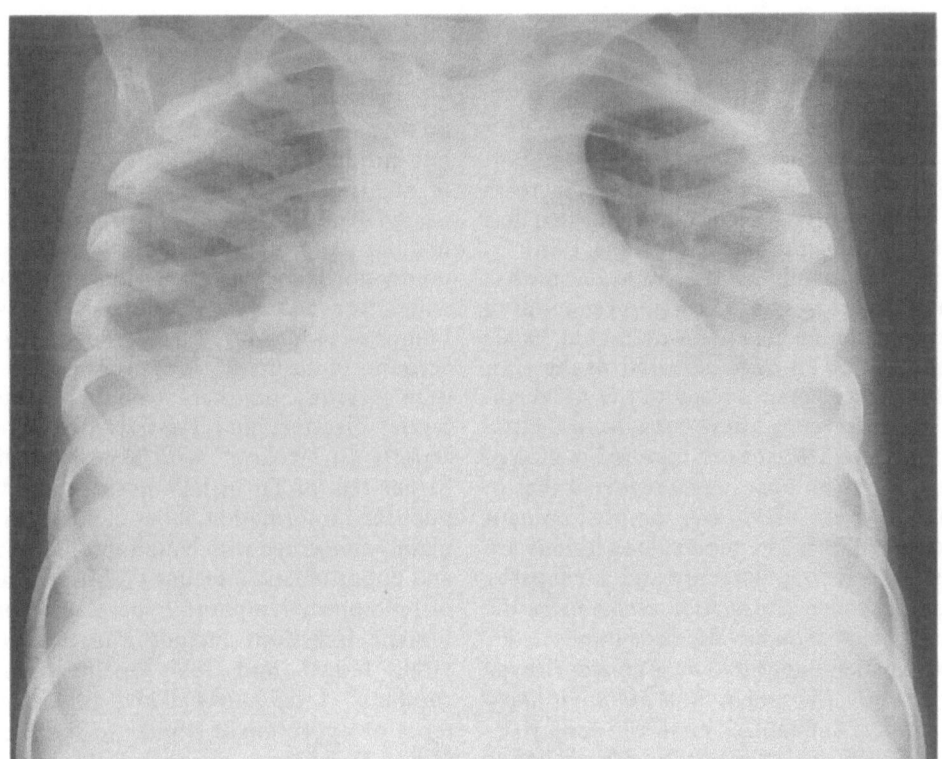

Fig. 3.49. CXR; bilateral chylothorax. Mediastinal and paratrachea widening from adenopathy. Pleural tap revealed chylous fluid. Mediastinal involvement of the thoracic duct is a rare occurrence in pulmonary TB.

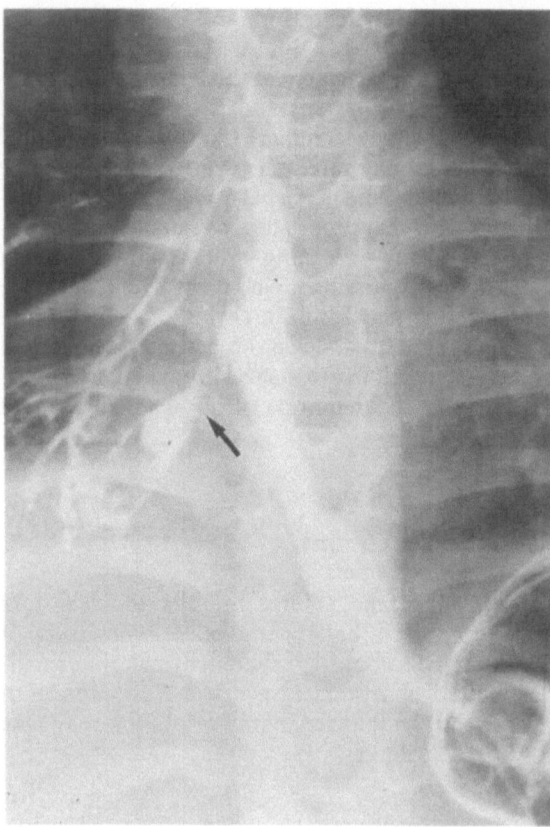

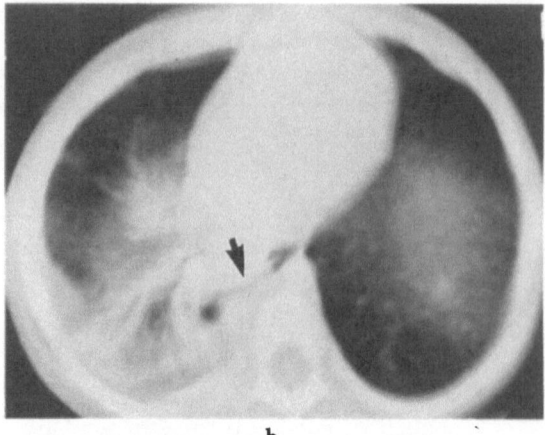

b

Fig. 3.50. a Barium swallow, b CT; broncho esophageal fistula is clearly shown (arrows). Histology at surgical resection confirmed a tract formed from TB mediastinal nodes.

a

HIV Infection

World-wide alarm has been caused by the increase of TB in HIV-positive serology patients that has been reported from Europe[33,34] and the USA[35-38]. These have been mainly adults and attention has been focused on urban slum areas, intravenous drug abusers and prison in-mates. An estimated 39,000 additional cases of TB have occurred in the USA between 1985 and 1991 as a result of the AIDS epidemic[39]. The worst reports have come from Central Africa[40,41] in which TB has been reported in 40% of AIDS patients. An autopsy series reported that in nearly 50% of severe AIDS cases the predominant pathology was MTB[42]. The tuberculous lesions are more likely to be extrapulmonary and adenopathy is a feature. Although reactivation seems to be the likely cause[38], reinfection has also been implicated[34]. HIV-positive patients appear to be at greater risk for acquiring primary TB[35] and in these cases it is likely to have a rapidly fulminating course[34]. In adult HIV-positive cases with bacteriologically proven active pulmonary TB, 10.5% of the CXRs were normal[37], but in others the infiltrates started in the superior segments of upper and lower lobes but rapidly appeared in all locations with a propensity for a coarse nodular pattern and glandular enlargement[38]. This is very much the appearance that we see in children with advanced primary progressive disease and an immuno-compromised background. There are few accounts in the literature of proven TB in AIDS children currently, but there is no doubt about the potential disasters and Central African experience reports an increase[43] with a possible eight times higher risk of TB in HIV-positive children[44]. The published information about children with AIDS is mainly concerned with lymphoproliferative diseases and opportunistic infections[45]. There is an increase of pulmonary lymphoid hyperplasia[46] and opportunistic infections include *Pneumocystis carinii*, viral, fungal and the *Mycobacterium avium* complex[47, 48] which may all give diffuse nodular patterns or appearances similar to those seen in TB (Figs 3.51, 3.52).

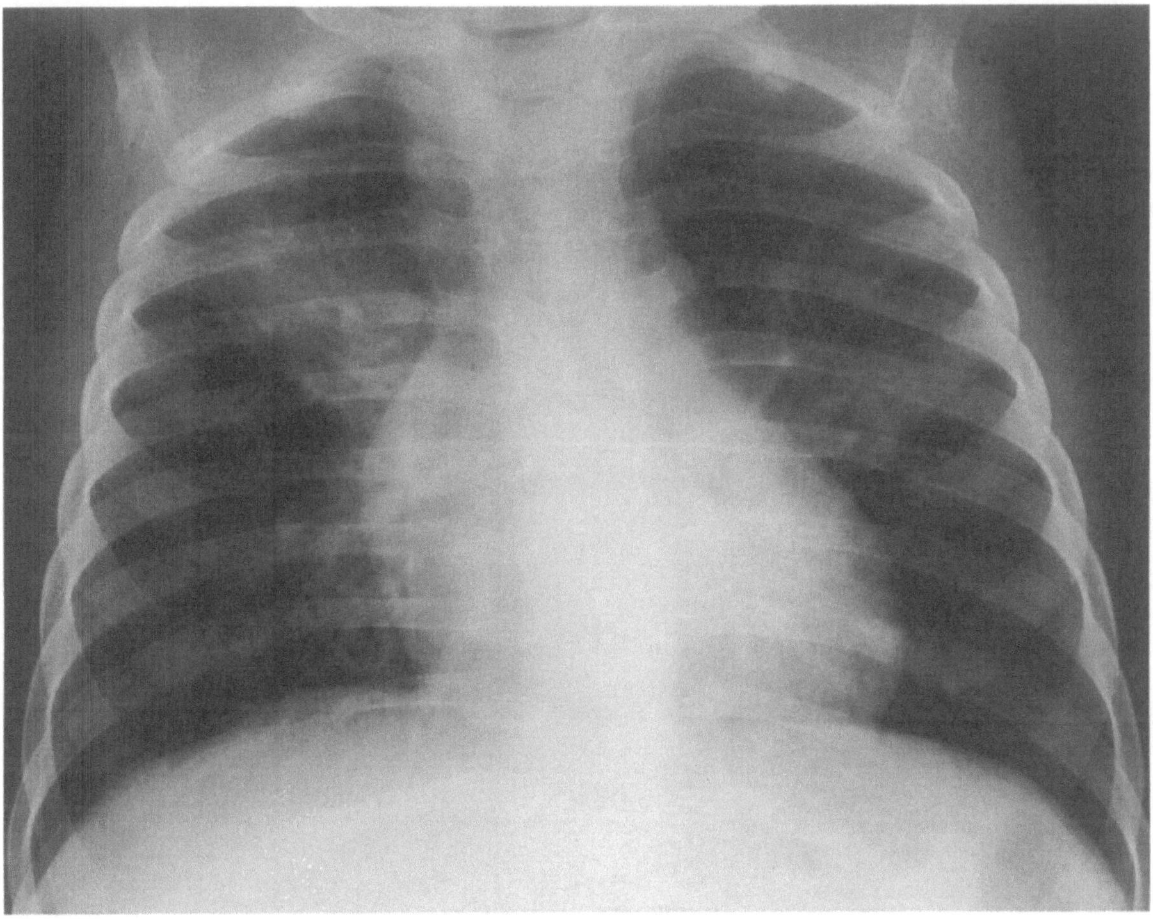

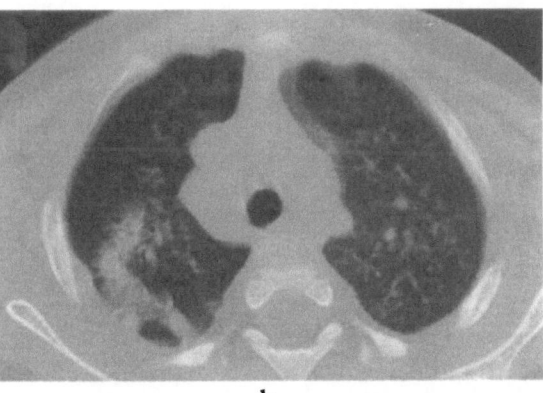

a

b

Fig. 3.51. a CXR, **b** CT; HIV-positive child RUL infiltrate and R paratracheal adenopathy could never be confirmed as TB skin testing and gastric washings/bronchial lavage were negative for TB. There was no response to anti-TB medication.

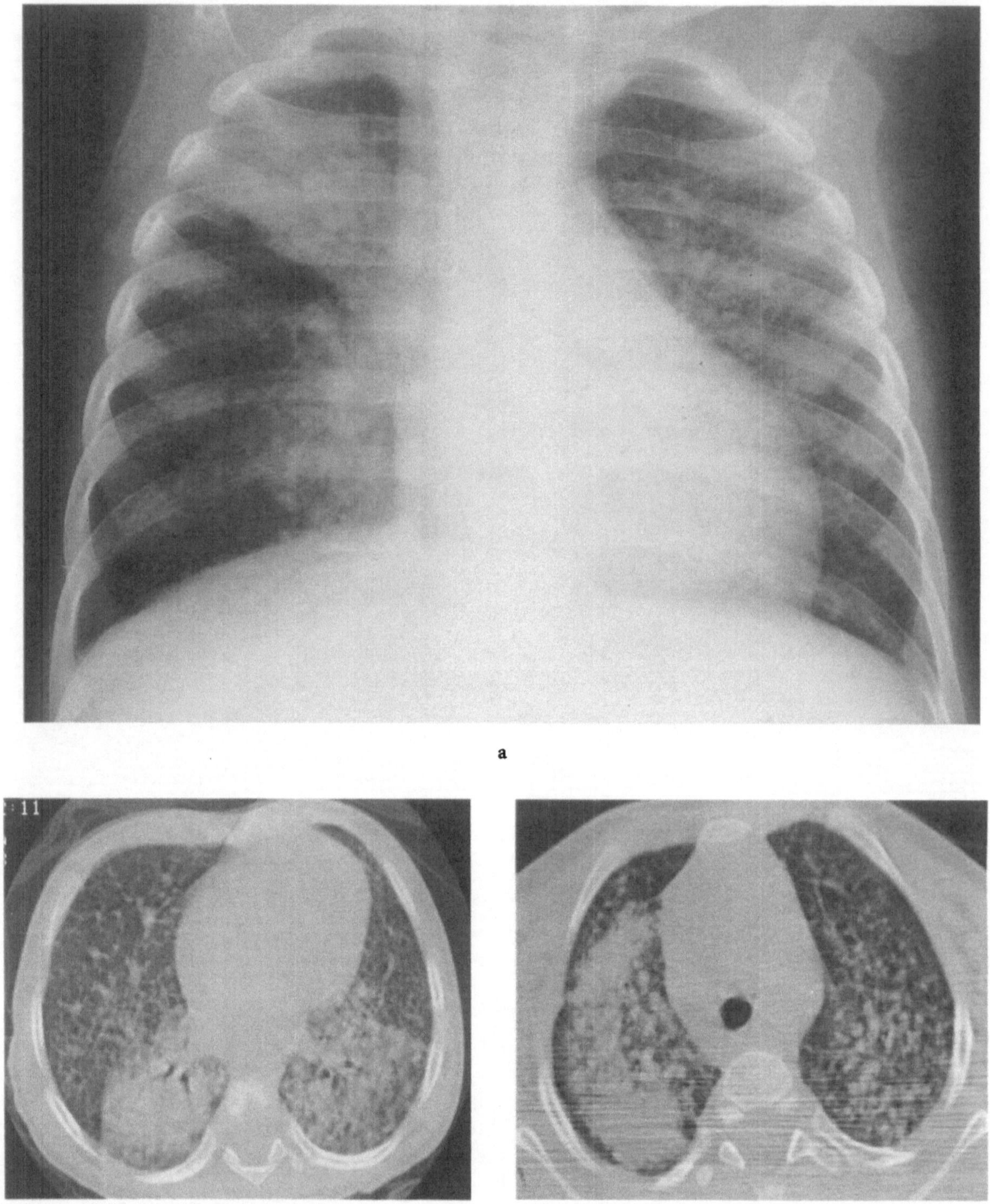

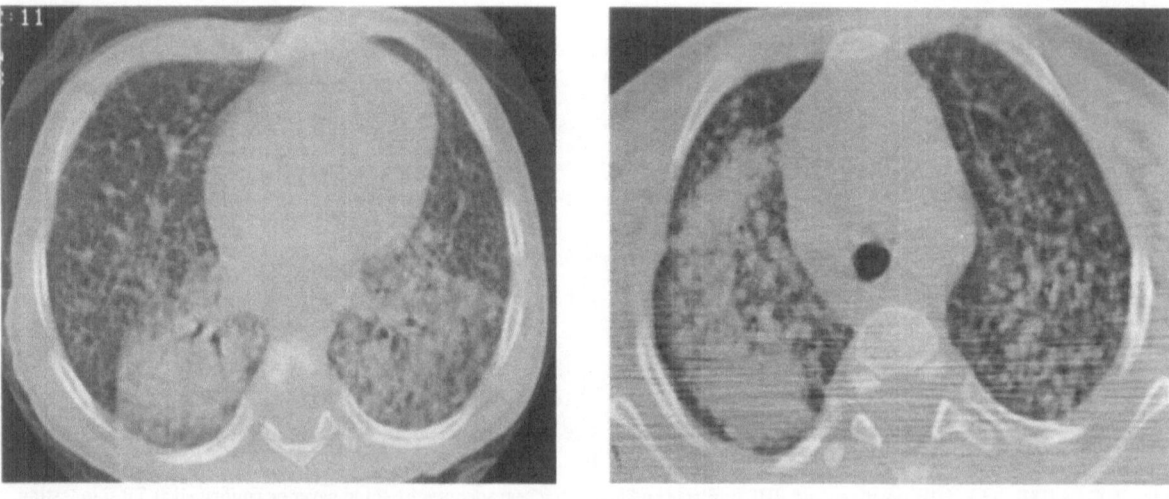

Fig. 3.52. a CXR, **b**,**c** CT; HIV-positive child. RUL, RLL, and more diffuse L parahilar infiltrates. R parahilar adenopathy was present. TB infection was never confirmed although improvement on anti-TB medication occurred.

References

1. Toman K (1976) Mass radiography in tuberculosis control. WHO Chronicle 30: 51-51
2. London RG (1979) Thoracic Tuberculosis: Clinical Aspects. Semin Roentgenol 14: 179-191
3. Amodio J, Abrahamson S, Berdon W (1986) Primary pulmonary tuberculosis: a resurgent disease in the urban United States. Pediatr Radiol 16: 185-189
4. Palmer PES (1979) Pulmonary tuberculosis - Usual and unusual radiographic presentations. Semin Roentgenol 14: 204-248
5. Bass JB, Farer LS, Hopewell PC, Jacobs RF, Snider DE (1990) Diagnostic standards and classification of tuberculosis. Am Rev Respir Dis 142: 725-735
6. Ghon A (1916) The Primary Lung Focus of Tuberculosis in Children. London, England: JA Churchill Ltd
7. Caffey J (1985) Primary Pulmonary Tuberculosis. In: Silverman F (ed) Pediatric X-Ray Diagnosis (8th ed). Chicago: IL Year Book, pp 1210-1227
8. Starke JR (1988) Modern approach to the diagnosis and treatment of tuberculosis in children. Pediatr Clin North Am 35: 441-464
9. Donald PR, Ball JB, Burger PJ (1985) Bacteriologically confirmed pulmonary tuberculosis in childhood. Clinical and radiological features. SAMJ 67: 588-590
10. Aderele WI (1980) Radiological patterns of pulmonary tuberculosis in Nigerian children. Tubercle 61: 157-163
11. Beyers JA (1991) Radiographic Manifestations. In: Coovadia HM, Benetar SR (Eds) A Century of Tuberculosis: South African Perspectives. Cape Town, South Africa: Oxford University Press, Ch 13, pp 203-223
12. Leung AN, Muller NL, Pineda PR, FitzGerald JM (1992) Primary tuberculosis in childhood: radiographic manifestations. Radiology 182: 87-91; and Pineda PR, Leung A, Muller NL, Allen EA, Black WA, FitzGerald JM (1993) Intrathoracic paediatric tuberculosis: a report of 202 cases. Tuberc Lung Dis 74: 261-266
13. Lamont AC, Cremin BJ, Pelteret RM (1986) Radiological patterns of pulmonary tuberculosis in the paediatric age group. Pediatr Radiol 16: 2-7
14. Weber AL, Bird KT, Janower ML (1966) Primary tuberculosis in children with particular emphasis on changes affecting the tracheobronchial tree. AJR 103: 123-132
15. Delacourt C, Mani TM, Bonnerot V, de Blic J, Sayec N, Lallemand D, Schienmann P (1993) Computed tomography with normal chest radiograph in tuberculous infection. Arch D Childhood 69: 430-432
16. Im J, Song KS, Kang HS, Park JH, Yeon KM, Han MC, Kim C (1987) Mediastinal tuberculous lymphadenitis: CT manifestations. Radiology 164: 115-119
17. Freiman I, Greefhuysen J, Solomon A (1975) The radiological presentation of pulmonary tuberculosis in children. SAMJ 49: 1703-1706
18. Im J, Itoh H, Shim YS, Lee JH, Ahn J, Han MC, Noma S (1993) Pulmonary tuberculosis, CT findings - early active disease and sequential changes with antituberculous therapy. Radiol 186: 653-660
19. Miller FJW (1982) Tuberculosis in children. Evolution, Epidemiology, Treatment and Prevention. Medicine in the Tropics. Edinburgh: Churchill Livingstone
20. Grenier P, Maurice F, Musset D, Menuj Y, Nahum H (1986) Bronchiectasis: assessment by thin-section CT1. Radiology 161: 95-99
21. McGuinness G, Naidich DP, Leithan BS, McCauley DI (1993) Bronchiectasis: CT Evaluation. AJR 160: 253-259
22. Jamieson DH, Cremin BJ (1993) High resolution CT of the lungs in acute disseminated tuberculosis and a pediatric radiology perspective of the term "miliary". Pediatr Radiol 23: 380-383
23. Hussey G, Chisholm T, Kibel M (1991) Miliary tuberculosis in children: a review of 94 cases. Paed Infect Dis J 10: 832-836
24. Glossary of terms of thoracic radiology: recommendations of the Fleischner Society. (1984) AJR 143: 509-517
25. Schuit KE (1979) Miliary tuberculosis in children. Clinical and laboratory manifestations in 19 patients. Am J Dis Child 133: 583-585
26. Aderle WI (1978) Miliary tuberculosis in Nigerian children. East Afr Med J 55: 166-171
27. Hugo-Hamman CT, Scher H, De Moor MMA (1994) Tuberculous pericarditis in children: a review of 44 cases. Pediatr Infect Dis J (1994) 13: 13-18
28. Polansky SM. Frank A, Ablow RC, Effmann EL (1978) Congenital Tuberculosis. Am J Roentgenol 130: 994-996
29. Nemir RL, O'Hare D (1985) Congenital tuberculosis. AJDC 139: 284-286
30. Bate TWP, Sinclair RE, Robinson MJ (1986) Neonatal tuberculosis. Arch Dis Childhood 61: 512-514
31. Schaaf HS, Gie RP, Beyers N, Smuts N, Donald PR (1993) Tuberculosis in infants less than 3 months of age. Arch D Child 69: 371-374
32. Agrons GA, Markowitz RI, Kramer SS (1993) Pulmonary tuberculosis in children. Semin Roengenol 28: 158-172
33. Goldman KP (1987) Editorial: AIDS and Tuberculosis. Br Med J 295: 511-512
34. Di Perri G, Danzi MC, de Checchi G et al. (1989) Nosocomial epidemic of active tuberculosis among HIV-infected patients. Lancet 2: 1502-1504
35. Sunderam G, McDonald RJ, Maniatis T et al. (1986) Tuberculosis as a manifestation of the acquired immunodeficiency syndrome (AIDS). JAMA 256: 362-366
36. Braun MM, Truman BI, Maguire B et al. (1989) Increasing incidence of tuberculosis in a prison inmate population. JAMA 26: 393-397
37. Fitzgerald JM, Grzybowski S, Allen EA (1991) The impact of human immunodeficiency virus on tuberculosis and its control. Chest 100: 191-200
38. Davis SD, Yankelevitz DF, Williams T, Henschke CI (1993) Pulmonary Tuberculosis in Immunocompromised Hosts: Epidemiological, Clinical, and Radiological Assessment. Semin Roentol 28: 119-130
39. MacGregor RR (1993) Tuberculosis: from history to current management. Semin Roentgenol 28: 101-108
40. Harries AD (1990) Tuberculosis and human immunodeficiency virus infection in developing countries. Lancet 335: 387-390
41. De Cock KM, Soro B, Coulibaly IM (1992) Tuberculosis and HIV infection in sub-Saharan Africa. JAMA 268: 1581-1587
42. Lucas SB, De Cock KM, Hounnou A et al. (1994) Contribution of tuberculosis in slim disease in Africa. Br Med J 308: 1531-1533
43. Chintu C, Bhat G, Luo C et al. (1993) Seroprevalence of human immunodeficiency virus type 1 infection in Zambian children with tuberculosis. Pediatr Infect Dis J 12: 499-504
44. Bhat GJ, Diwan VK, Chintu C, Kabika M, Masona J (1993) HIV, BCGT and TB in Children: A Case Control Study in Lusaka, Zambia. J Tropical Pediatr 39: 219-223
45. Haller JO, Cohen HL (1994) Pediatric HIV infection: an imaging update. Pediatr Radiol 24: 224-230
46. Connor EM, Marquis J, Oleske JM (1991) Lymphoid interstitial pneumonitis. In: Pizzo PA, Wilfert CM (Eds) Pediatric

AIDS: The challenge of HIV infection in infants, children and adolescents. Williams & Wilkins, Baltimore: pp 343–353

47. Horsburgh CR, Caldwell MB, Simonds RJ (1993) Epidemiology of disseminated nontuberculous mycobacterial disease in children with acquired immunodeficiency syn-

drome. Pediatr Infect Dis 12: 219–221

48. Berdon WE, Mellins R, Abramson SJ et al. (1993) Pediatric HIV infection in the second decade: the changing pattern of lung involvement (clinical and plain film and CT findings). Radiol Clin North Am 31: 453–463

4 Imaging of Central Nervous System Tuberculosis

D.H. Jamieson and B.J. Cremin

Imaging Methods

1. *Computed Tomography (CT)*
   CT is the essential imaging modality for evaluation for intracranial disease. Maximal information is obtained from studies without and with intravenous contrast enhancement.

2. *Magnetic Resonance Imaging (MR)*
   MR is the imaging modality of choice. Availability and expense restrict its universal use. Gadolinium enhancement is a very useful adjunct.

3. *Ultrasound (US)*
   US can readily detect hydrocephalus but it is of little practical use as TB involvement is rare under 6 months of age when fontanelle access is good.

4. *Plain films*
   Plain films are of little practical use in modern imaging. Basal or tuberculoma calcification may be seen and splayed sutures indicate established hydrocephalus.

The CNS parenchyma is involved secondarily to hematogenous spread of bacilli. Meningeal disease follows rupture of an ependymal-based granuloma into the subarachnoid space[1], rupture of an intimal granuloma in a vessel related to the subarachnoid space or, rarely, contiguous spread from a TB osteitis (e.g. mastoiditis).

The pathology can be divided into TB meningitis and its sequelae, and granulomatous mass lesions, both parenchymal and meningeal. When granulomatous lesions are of tuberculous etiology they may be referred to as tuberculomas.

Tuberculous Meningitis (TBM)

TBM is responsible for the most serious morbidity and mortality of TB infection, and early diagnosis and treatment offers the single best chance of a good prognosis[2]. The clinical presentation can be insidious with lethargy, vomiting, loss of weight and irritability preceding meningism. The severity of the disease on presentation has been classified as[3]:

Stage 1; fully conscious, meningeal irritation and no focal signs

Stage 2; mental confusion with cranial nerve lesion or hemiparesis

Stage 3; comatose with or without hemiplegia.

The association of TBM with progressive primary pulmonary disease or acute hematogenous dissemination is high, up to 90%[4]. The cerebrospinal fluid (CSF) is usually clear with, classically, a relatively low cell count, elevated lymphocytes, elevated protein and reduced chloride and glucose levels. However, increased cell counts with polymorphonuclear predominance, normal glucose and decreased protein can occur, causing diagnostic problems with viral and bacterial infections[5].

There are no defense mechanisms in the subarachnoid space to impede the spread of the early exudative phase of the infection. A granulomatous inflammatory response develops in the basal cisterns with a thick gelatinous exudate. Extension along cerebral vessels and up to the convexity may occur. The proliferative inflammatory reaction shows microscopic granuloma formation and is

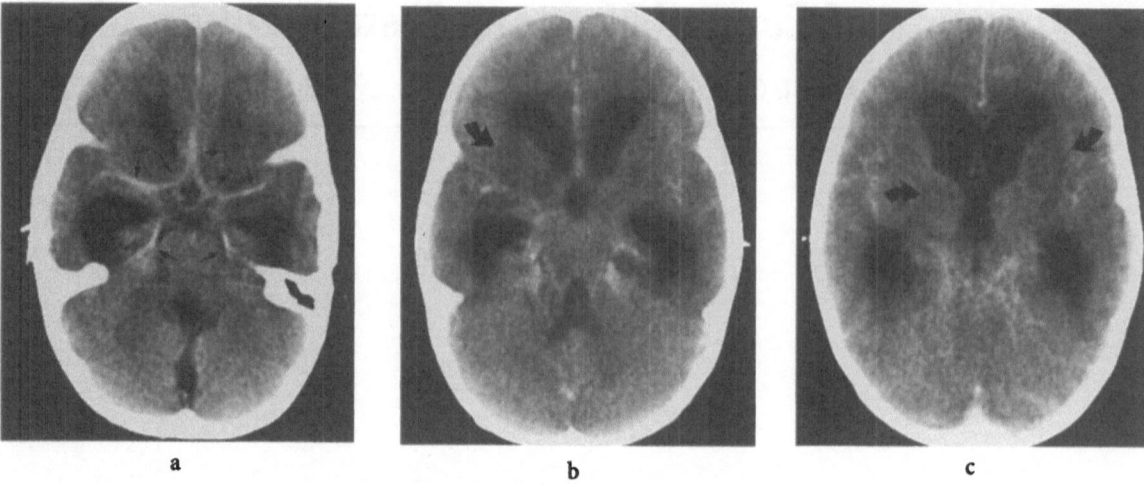

Fig. 4.1a–c.   IV contrast-enhanced CT: tuberculous menigitis; the triad of basal leptomeningeal enhancement (small arrows), infarction in the basal ganglia (curved arrows) and hydrocephalus is present.

responsible for the basal enhancement seen on intravenous (IV) contrast-enhanced CT and IV gadolinium-enhanced MR studies (Figs 4.1, 4.2, 4.3).

Vasculitis and obstruction to the flow of CSF cause the most damaging sequelae of TBM.

The incidence of infarction of TBM is between 40% and 60%[6,7]. Blood vessels traversing the proliferative arachnoiditis become involved, and vasculitis, spasm and occlusion result in infarction[8]. The penetrating arteries to the brain stem and basal ganglia are most affected. In early infarction, CT

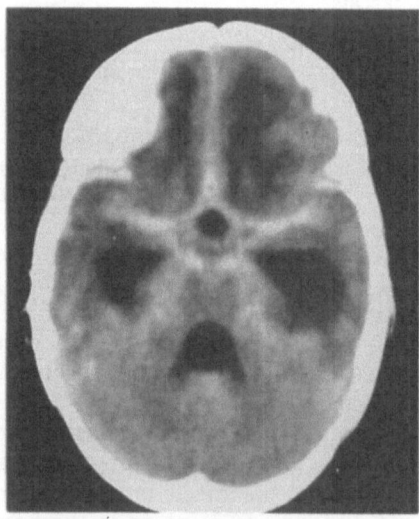

Fig. 4.2.   IV contrast-enhanced CT: tuberculous meningitis; florid basal enhancement and hydrocephalus.

shows ill-defined hypodense areas, mass effect may be detected and variable peripheral, sometimes diffuse, IV contrast enhancement occurs (Figs 4.4, 4.5). This progresses to a well-defined hypodense lesion (Fig. 4.6). MR is far superior to CT in accessing the extent and anatomic location of the infarcts, particularly in the brain stem. A recent infarct is a T2 hyperintense lesion which may show mass effect and have variable IV gadolinium enhancement (Fig. 4.7). There is progression to a well-defined T1 hypointense, T2 hyperintense cavitated infarct (Fig 4.3a). Infarction of major vessels can occur with complete vascular territory involvement (Fig. 4.8) and the end result of infarction can be extensive encephalomalacia (Fig. 4.9).

The proliferative arachnoiditis can obstruct the normal flow of CSF from the choroid plexus to the arachnoid granulations on the convexity. The resultant hydrocephalus is the most constant finding in TB meningitis (Figs 4.1–4.9)[9,10]. The block is usually extraventricular in the region of the basal cisterns; however, an aqueduct obstruction, identified by acutely dilated lateral and third ventricles and small fourth ventricle, is occasionally noted (Fig. 4.10). This is an important finding as these patients require immediate shunt procedures. The chronic phase of TBM, which may be related to antituberculous therapy, results in fibrosis of arachnoid tissues[8]. This may continue to obstruct the basal cisterns and cause persistence of hydrocephalus (Figs 4.9, 4.11).

Progressive fibrotic changes may affect blood vessels, with narrowing and even occlusion.

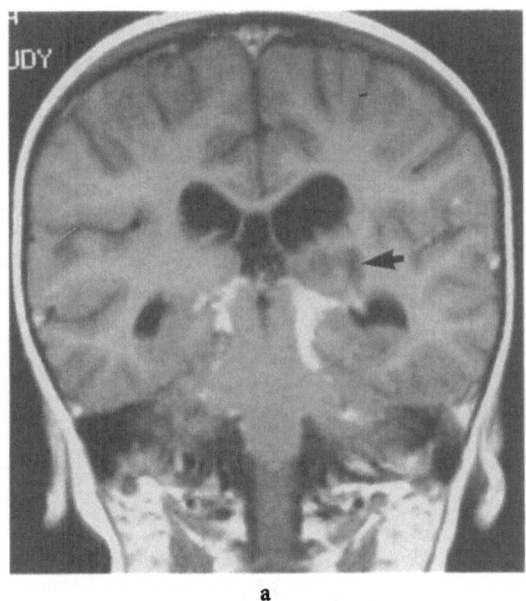 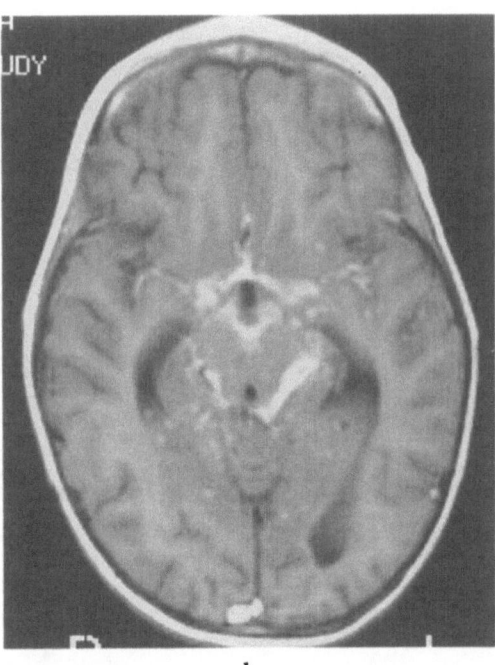

a   b

Fig. 4.3. **a** Coronal and **b** axial IV gadolinium-enhanced T1 MR: tuberculous meningitis; the triad with basal leptomeningeal enhancement, cavitated infarct in the L deep grey matter (arrow) and hydrocephalus. Note the size of the left ambient cistern lesion in keeping with progression to a meningeal granuloma.

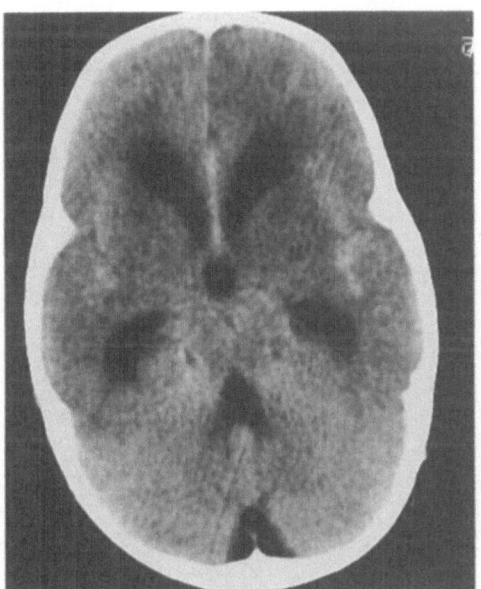 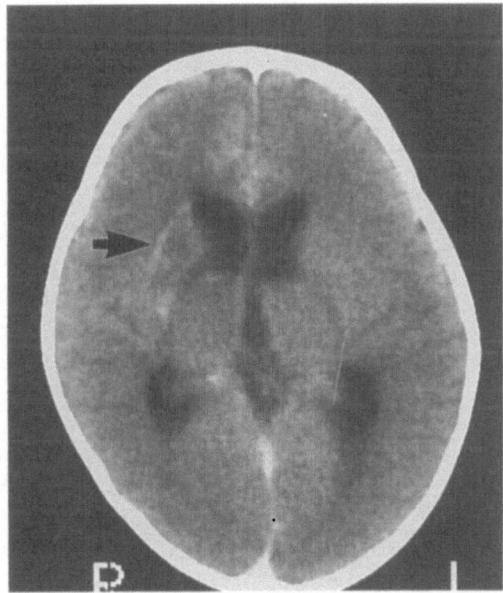

Fig. 4.4. IV contrast-enhanced CT: tuberculous meningitis; bilateral early basal ganglia infarction shows hypodense changes with no enhancement and minimal mass effect.

Fig. 4.5. IV contrast-enhanced CT: tuberculous meningitis; peripheral enhancing R caudate head infarct (arrow).

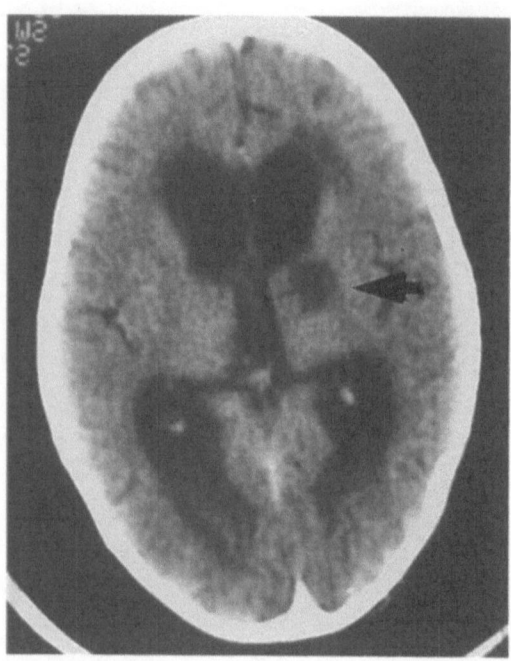

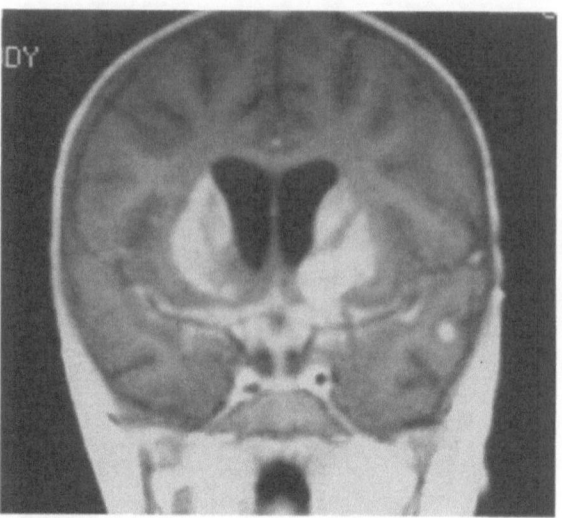

Fig. 4.7. Coronal IV gadolinium-enhanced T1 MR: tuberculous meningitis; leptomeningeal enhancement of suprasellar cistern and following both middle meningeal vessels is well shown. There are bilateral enhancing infarcts in the basal ganglia and hydrocephalus.

Fig. 4.6. IV contrast-enhanced CT: tuberculous meningitis; hydrocephalus and well-defined low density old L deep grey matter infarct (arrow).

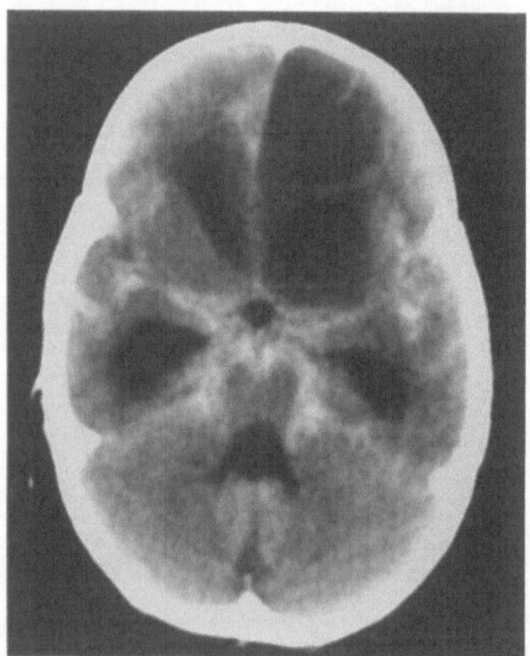

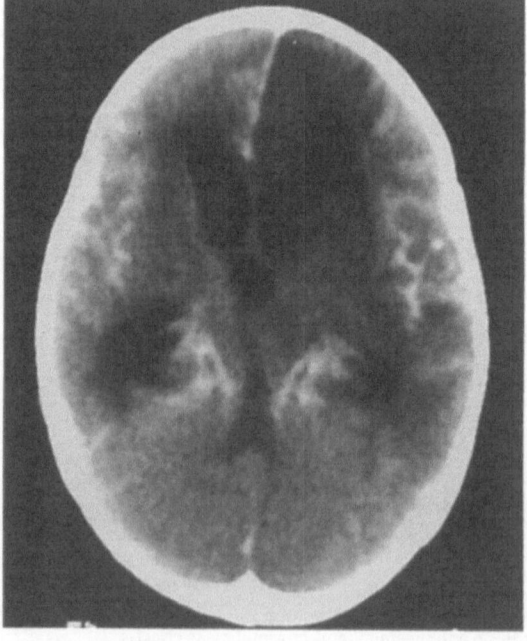

a

b

Fig. 4.8a,b. IV contrast-enhanced CT: tuberculous meningitis; there is basal leptomeningeal enhancement, hydrocephalus and infarction of the left anterior cerebral artery territory.

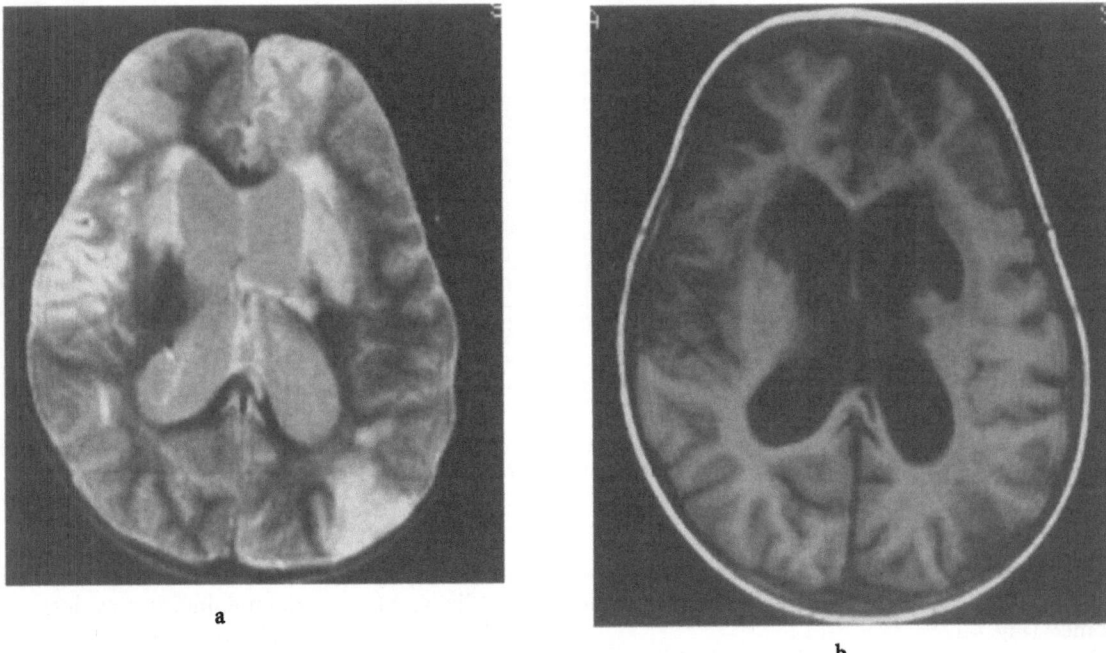

Fig. 4.9. a Axial T2 and **b** axial T1 MR: sequelae of tuberculous meningitis; ventricles remain dilated, there is T2 hyperintense, T1 hypointense encephalomalacia of the cortex and in the basal ganglia following infarction.

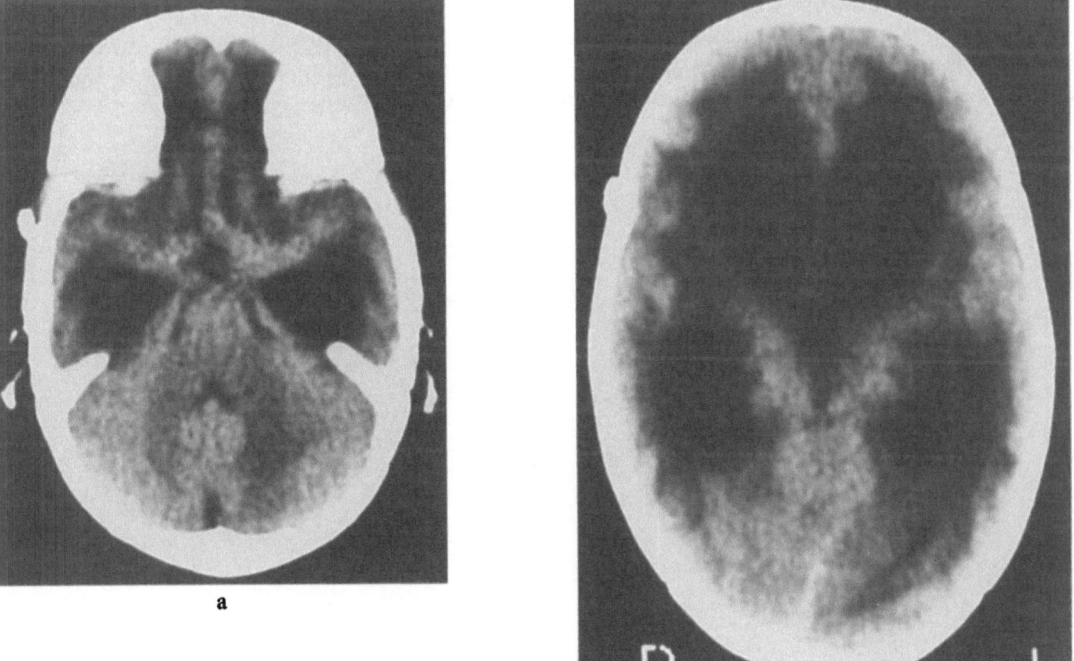

Fig. 4.10a,b. CT: tuberculous meningitis; periventricular hypodense change indicates acute dilation of the lateral ventricles and third ventricle and lack of dilation of the fourth ventricle indicates aqueduct obstruction.

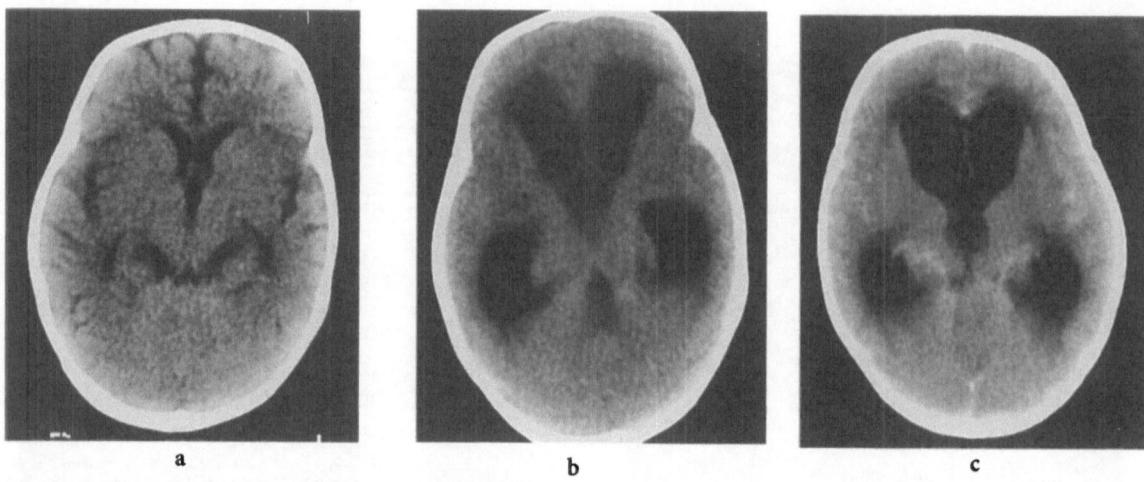

a   b   c

Fig. 4.11a–c. CT: these three studies show the persistence and progression of hydrocephalus in a patient with tuberculous meningitis on treatment. **a** on admission, **b** after 1 month and **c** 3 months later.

Involvement of carotid vessels as they traverse the meninges may be a rare cause of moya-moya syndrome[11] (Fig. 4.12).

Cranial nerves traversing the basal cisterns, in particular II, VI and VII, are often affected, with resultant palsy.

A triad in TBM that consists of basal contrast enhancement, hydrocephalus and infarction, has been reported in the literature[6,12,13]. Unfortunately, when present, the child is invariably neurologically compromised. Profound basal leptomeningeal enhancement is characteristic; however, it is variable and may not be prominent even in confirmed TB meningitis (Fig. 4.13). Bacterial meningitis may, less commonly, cause both some moderate basal contrast enhancement and a hydrocephalus which may be persistent; however, the hydrocephalus is more often transient and not persistent as it is in TB meningitis. A rare but important consideration in the differential diagnosis of TBM is a diffuse meningeal malignancy, such as may occur in medulloblastoma. Sarcoidosis is rare in children and the suspicion of a fungal meningitis is increased in immune-compromised patients.

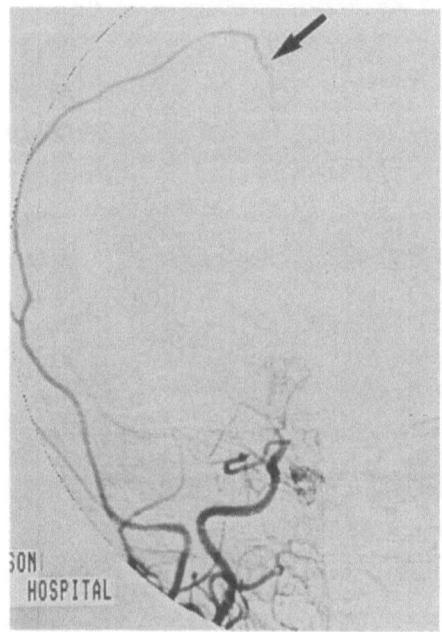

a

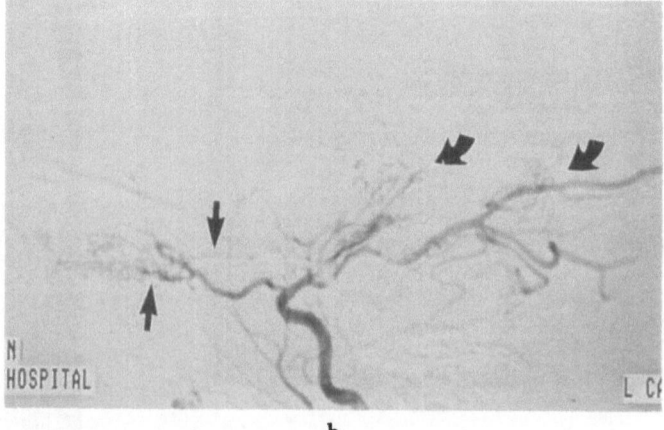

b

Fig. 4.12a,b. R carotid angiogram **a** AP and **b** lateral: moya-moya syndrome; there is near complete occlusion of the carotid vessel as it traverses the meninges. Colateral vascular supply has been taken from the middle meningeal artery (long arrows), the ophthalmic artery (short arrows) and from posterior circulation (curved arrrows).

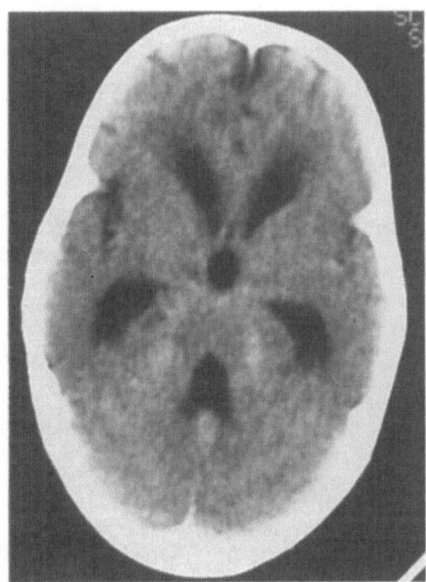

Fig. 4.13. IV contrast-enhanced CT: tuberculous meningitis; study done on clinical presentation shows little basal leptomeningeal enhancement and hydrocephalus.

Parenchymal Granulomatous Mass Lesions

About 10% of TB meningitis children have detected tuberculomas (Fig. 4.14), but the commonest presentation of tuberculomas is with a focal seizure. They vary in size from 0.5 cm to 3 cm but may be occasionally larger, up to 6 cm. They are often single (Fig. 4.15) but 15%–20% have multiple lesions (Fig. 4.16) and grape-like clusters of tuberculomas may occur (Fig. 4.17). Tuberculomas have a tendency to be peripheral but may occur anywhere in the parenchyma.

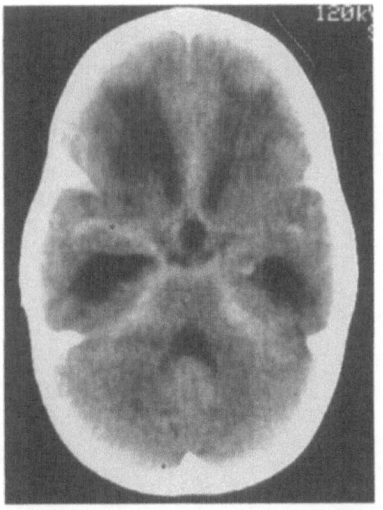

a

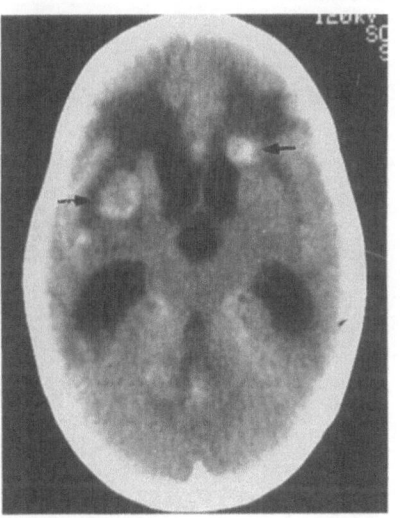

b

Fig. 4.14a,b. IV contrast-enhanced CT: tuberculous meningitis; basal enhancement and hydrocephalus is associated with parenchyma granulomas (arrows).

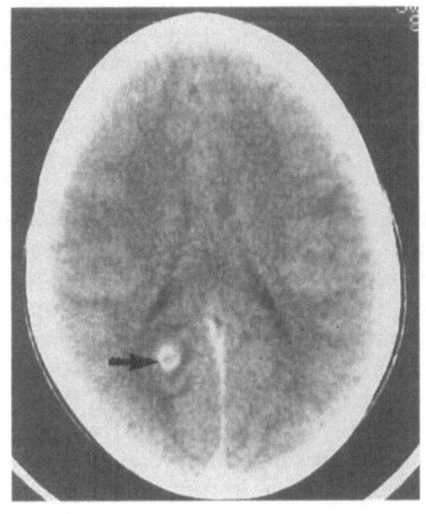

a

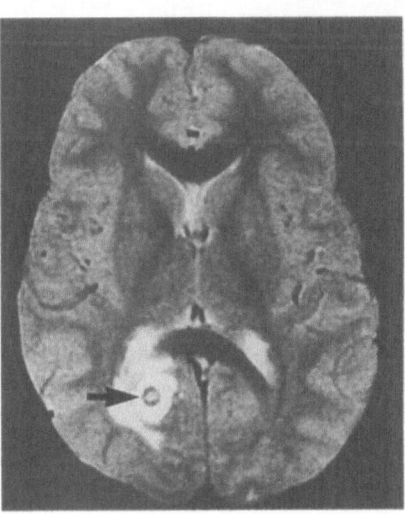

b

Fig. 4.15. **a** IV contrast-enhanced CT and **b** T2 MR: caseous tuberculoma; **a** contrast enhancing granuloma has a hypodense centre and hypodense surrounding vasogenic edema (arrow), **b** caseous necrotic centre is T2 hyperintense, the granuloma rim T2 hypointense (arrow) and the vasogenic edema T2 hyperintense.

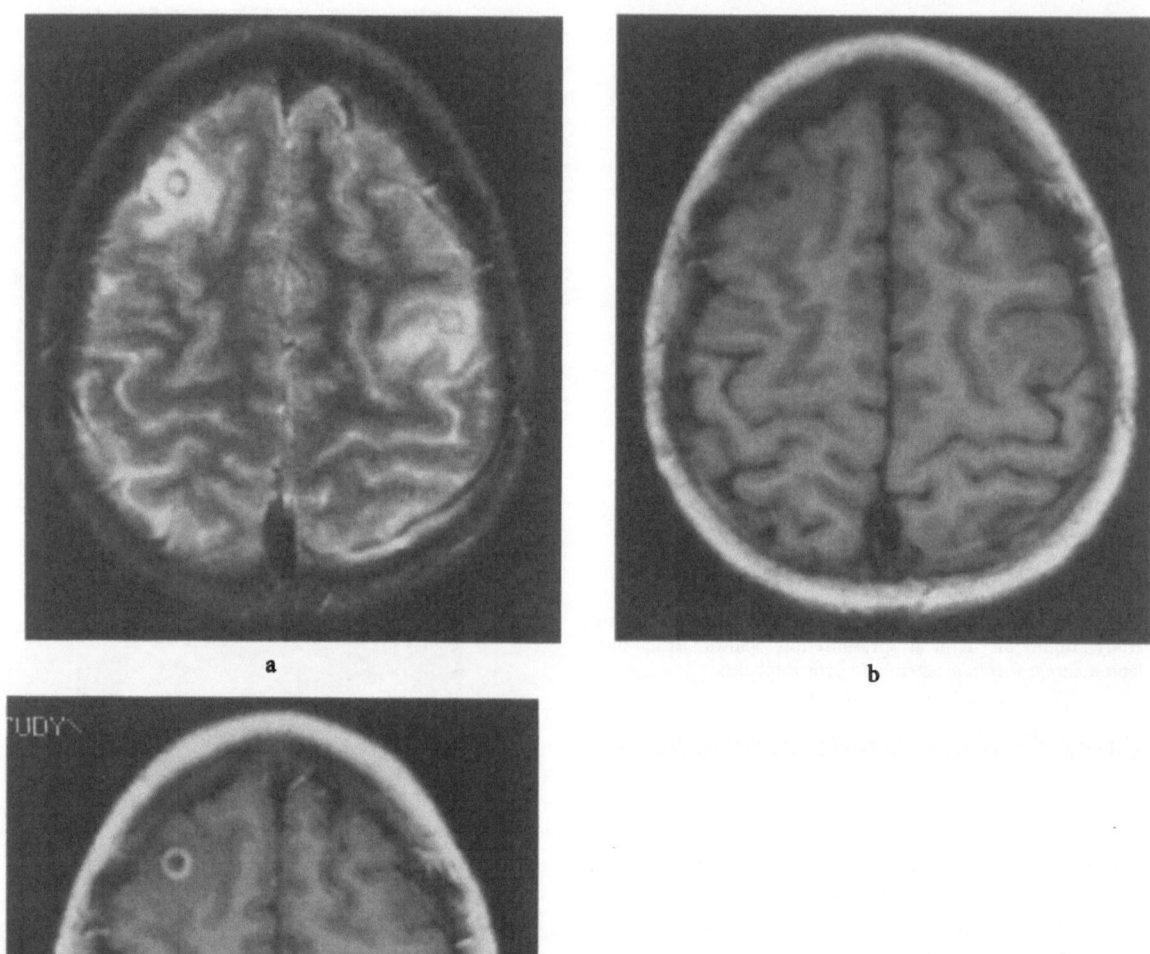

Fig. 4.16a–c. Axial MR: caseous tuberculomas; **a** T2 MR shows T2 hyperintense vasogenic edema, T2 hypointense granuloma rims and T2 hyperintense caseous necrotic centres, **b** T1 MR, shows vasogenic edema is hypointense and poorly demonstrated, the granuloma rims are slightly hyperintense and the caseous necrotic centres are hypointense, **c** IV gadolinium-enhanced MR demonstrates marked granuloma rim enhancement.

Symptomatic tuberculomas have surrounding vasogenic edema. This is hypodense on CT and T2 hyperintense on MR, with the characteristic inter-digitating pattern of white matter involvement. The edema does not enhance following IV contrast administration (Figs 4.15, 4.16).

A tuberculoma without macroscopic necrosis is iso to hyperdense on CT. MR shows slight T1 hyper-intensity and marked T2 signal shortening giving hypointensity. There is uniform enhancement fol-

lowing IV contrast medium on CT and IV gadolinium on MR (Fig. 4.18). However, central necrosis is usual in tuberculomas and this necrosis does not enhance, so that an enhancing ring lesion develops.

It is not commonly known that two necrotic processes occur in these granulomas. Both appear similar macroscopically, and microscopically with H & E staining and only the use of silver (reticulin) stains separates the two necrotic processes[14]. The commonest necrotic process in confirmed tubercu-

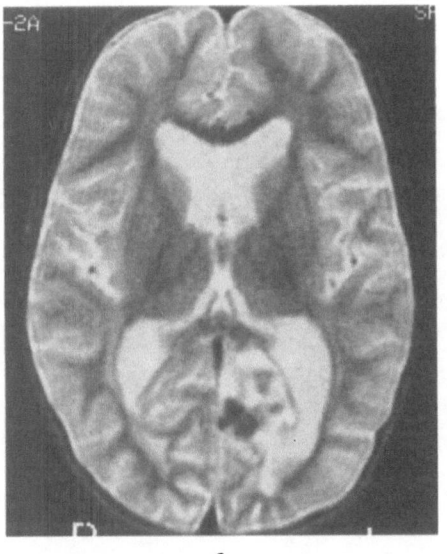

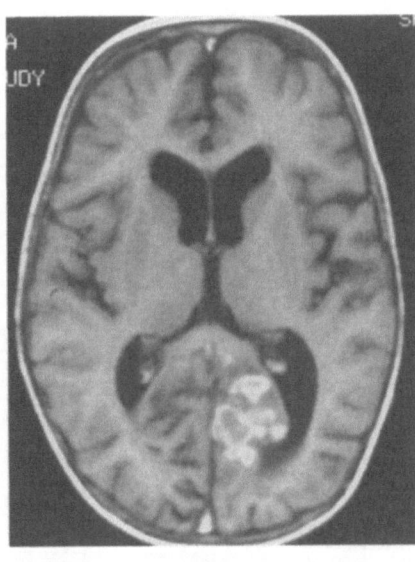

Fig. 4.17a,b. Axial MR: **a** T2, **b** IV gadolinium-enhanced T1: a grape-like cluster of granulomas is demonstrated in the L occipital lobe.

a

b

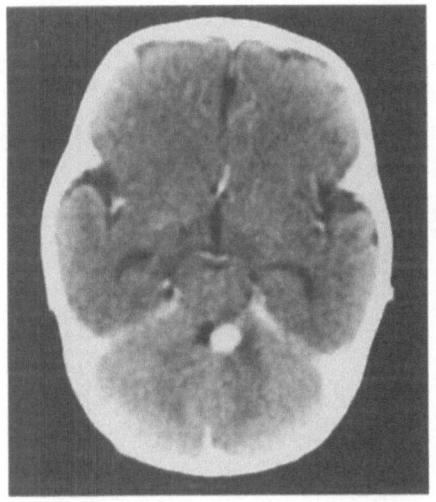

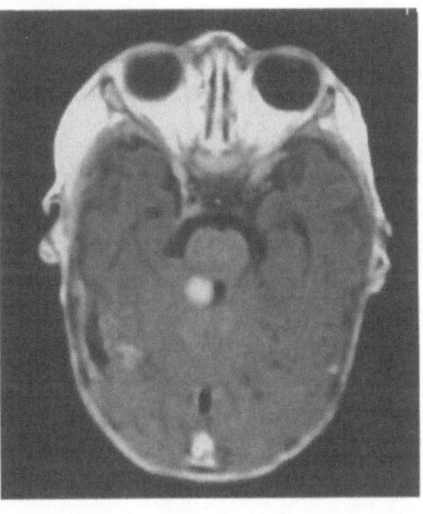

Fig. 4.18. **a** CT IV contrast-enhanced **b** MR IV gadolinium-enhanced T1: the uniform enhancing granuloma indicates no macroscopic evidence of necrosis.

a

b

loma is a gummatous necrosis where the inflammatory granulation tissue itself undergoes necrosis. This can occur intermittently, forming layers or a lamellated lesion. The necrotic region of these gummatous granulomas is iso to hyperdense on CT, and T1 isointense, T2 hypointense on MR and does not contrast enhance (Figs 4.17, 4.19, 4.20, 4.21). They are often 2 cm or larger on presentation.

The second necrotic process results from necrosis of a purely cellular infiltrate with no fibrovascular stroma identifiable on silver staining. This cellular infiltrate may have a variable component of epithelioid cells, macrophages and polymorphonucleocytes. Its consistency can vary from inspissated and "caseous" to liquefied and "abscess like". A higher concentration of polymorphonucleocytes is associated with more liquefied or pus-like content[14]. The central necrotic region of caseating granulomas or granulomatous abscesses is hypodense on CT and T1 isointense, T2 hyperintense on MR with no contrast enhancement (Figs 4.15, 4.16). These lesions are usually under 2 cm although large tuberculous abscesses may rarely occur (Fig. 4.22).

Both necrotic processes may be present in the same lesion in variable combinations (Fig. 4.23).

Tuberculomas resolve in 3–6 months on treatment for TB, but large lesions may take considerably longer. However, isolated tuberculomas may resolve without treatment and a minority (1%–5%) may calcify. Paradoxically, the appearance of new

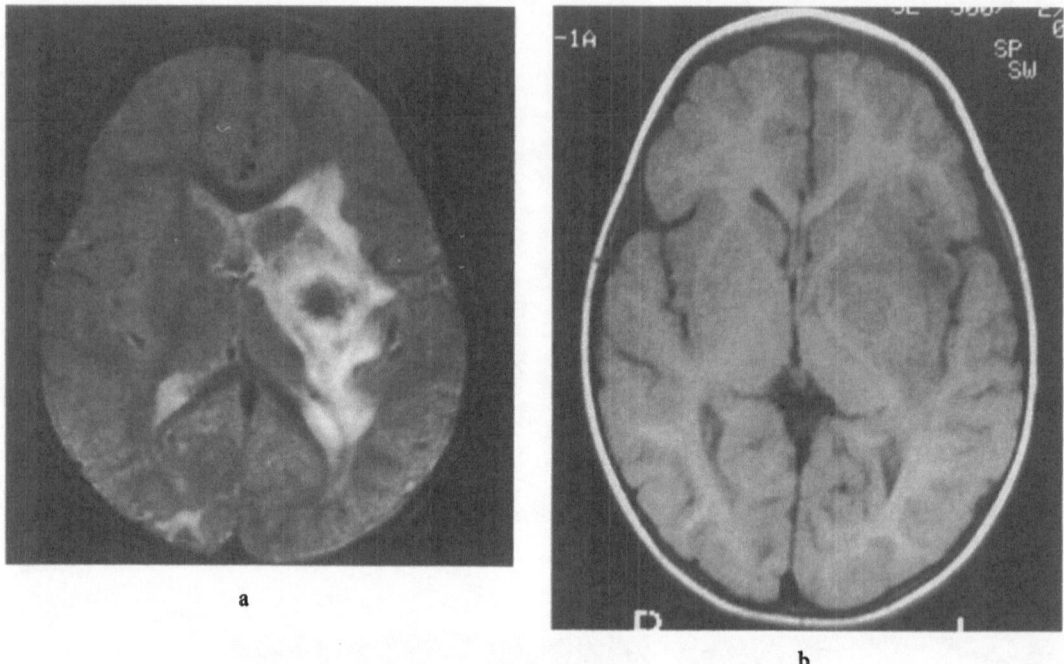

Fig. 4.19a,b. Axial MR: **a** T2, **b** T1: gummatous tuberculoma; T2 hyperintense vasogenic edema surrounds a predominantly T2 hypointense granuloma, T1 findings show the lesion to be T1 isointense.

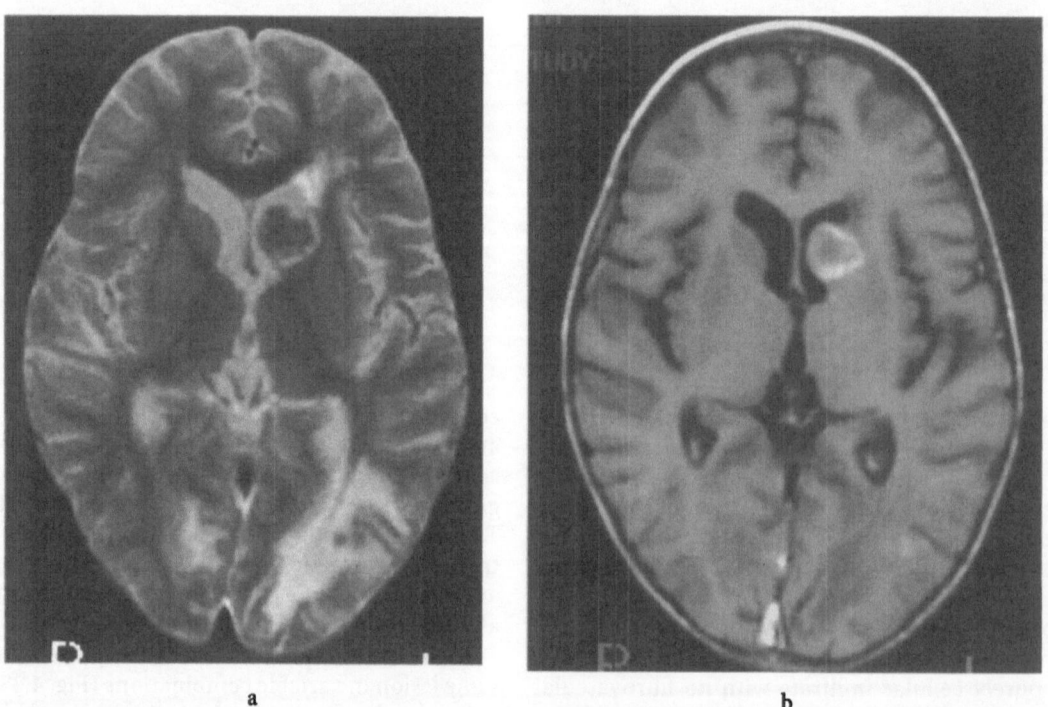

Fig. 4.20a,b. Axial MR: **a** T2, **b** IV gadolinium T1: gummatous tuberculoma; large left caudate head lesion is T2 hypointense with peripheral gadolinium enhancement. The central necrotic area does not enhance. Note a smaller L occipital granuloma with marked vasogenic edema.

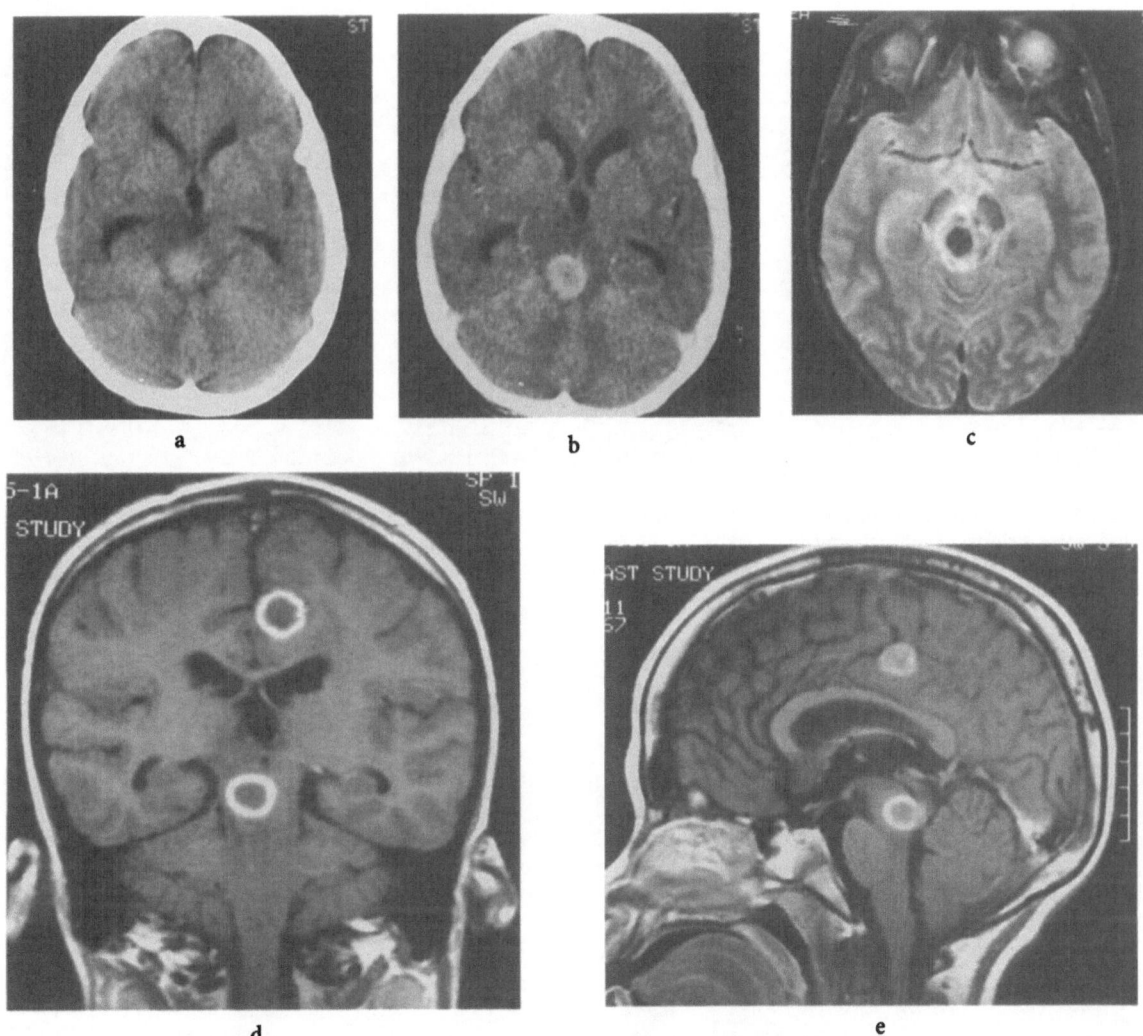

Fig. 4.21a–e. Gummatous tuberculomas: **a,b**: axial unenhanced and IV contrast-enhanced CT: large midbrain lesion is hyper-dense with irregular peripheral enhancement, **c** axial T2 MR, **d** coronal IV gadolinium-enhanced MR, **e** sagittal IV gadolinium-enhanced MR: the gummatous necrosis shows T2 hypointensity and the gadolinium studies show strong rim enhancement; note the well-demonstrated second gummatous tuberculoma in the parafalcine L parietal lobe.

granulomas or an increase in size of granulomas in patients on anti-TB therapy may also occur (Fig. 4.24) but is uncommon.

Although, theoretically, syphilis may require exclusion, MR allows a reasonable diagnosis of tuberculous etiology in the gummatous type of granulomas in children. The T2 hyperintense centre of the mass lesion will usually exclude tumor from the differential diagnosis. However the imaging features of the caseating granuloma or granulomatous abscess are not specific for TB and are indistinguishable from cysticercus granuloma or fungal and pyogenic lesions[14]. In areas where both TB and cysticercosis are prevalent the etiology of a single ring-enhancing lesion detected on CT in a patient investigated for a focal or generalised seizure remains a diagnostic dilemma[15], as imaging cannot distinguish between a caseating tuberculoma, a cysticercosis granuloma or a fungal lesion. At the Red Cross Children's Hospital in Cape Town, the policy is influenced by the high incidence of TB infection in the community and all children with lesions suspicious of tuberculoma are put on to anti-TB treatment even though similar lesions (and even tuberculomas) may resolve without treatment[16,17,18].

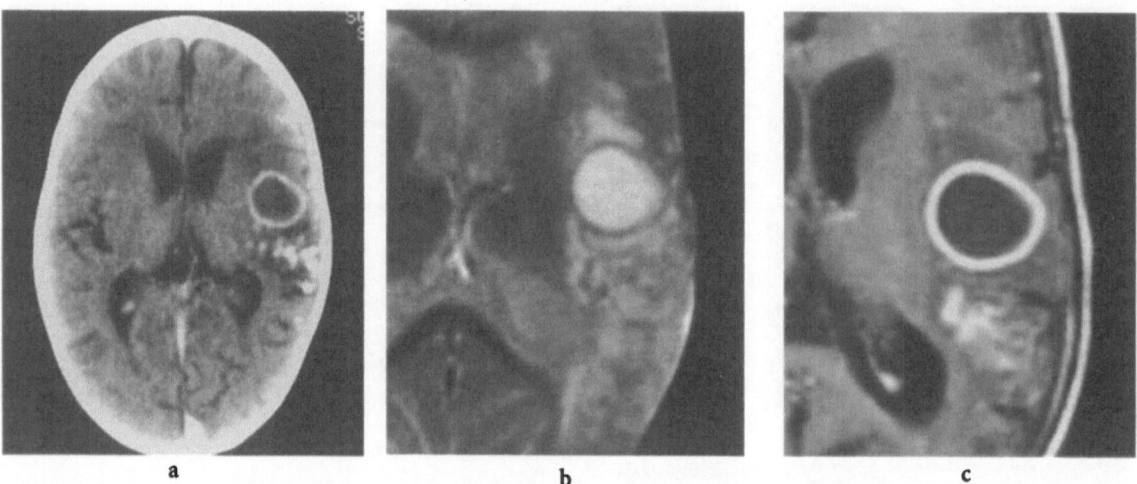

Fig. 4.22a–c. Tuberculous abscess: **a** IV contrast-enhanced CT demonstrates large L parietal ring enhancing lesion with a hypodense centre, a cluster of enhancing meningocerebral granulomas are noted posterior to this. **b** Axial T2 MR. T2 hypointense rim and T2 hyperintense centre is noted. **c** Axial IV gadolinium-enhanced T1 MR: enhancement of the abscess wall and the posterior meningocerebral granulomas are shown. Abscess content is T1 hypointense.

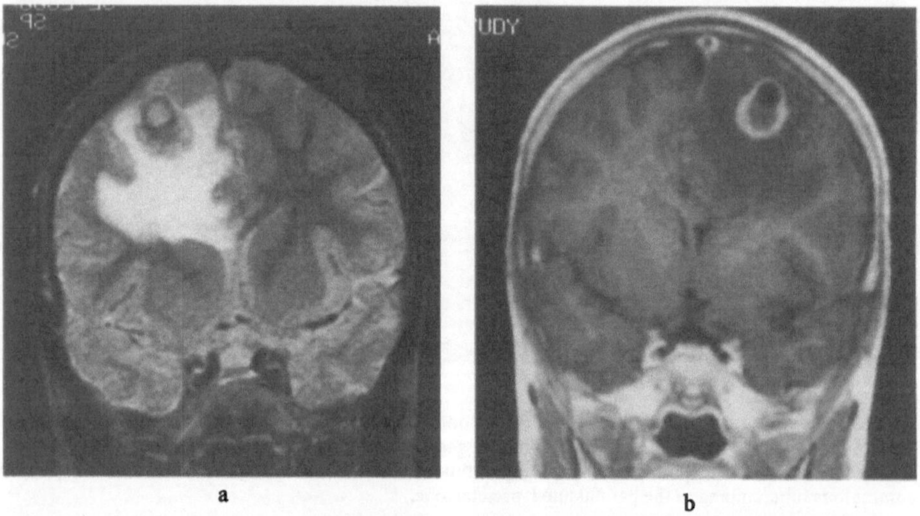

Fig. 4.23a,b. Coronal MR: **a** T2, **b** IV gadolinium-enhanced T1: mixed granuloma; the enhancing granuloma demonstrates a T1 hypointense, T2 hyperintense upper component (caseous necrosis) and a T1 isointense T2 hypointense lower component (gummatous necrosis).

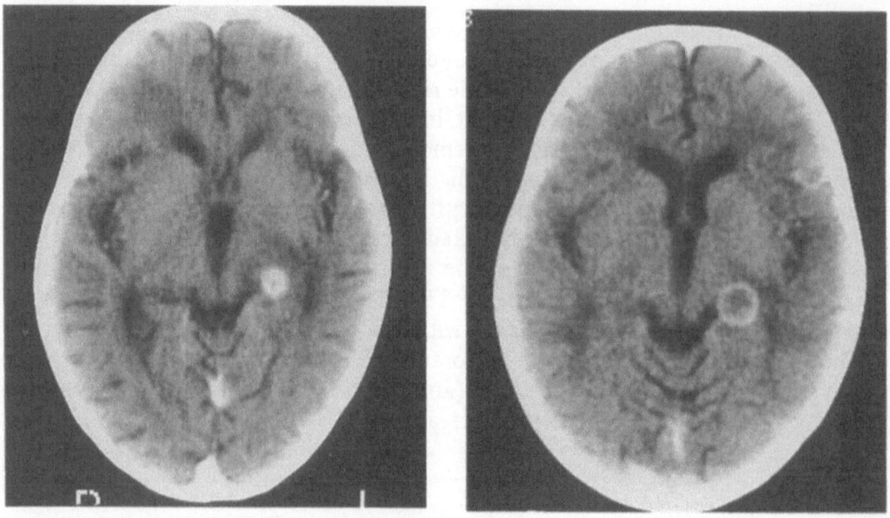

Fig. 4.24a,b. IV contrast-enhanced CT: tuberculoma enlargement on treatment: **a** scan on admission and **b** scan repeated after 4 months of appropriate antituberculous therapy with increased size.

Meningeal and Meningocerebral Granulomatous Mass Lesions

The proliferative arachnoiditis of a TB meningitis can progress to localized granuloma formation. Areas of predilection are the suprasellar and ambient cisterns (Figs 4.25, 4.26), but occurrence throughout the subarachnoid space can occur. Meningeal granulomas may be large enough to display mass effect and cause edema in adjacent parenchyma. Although the proliferative component predominates in the meningeal granuloma, gummatous and caseous/liquifactive necrosis can occur[14]. Imaging characteristics of the meningeal granulomas are the same as parenchymal lesions with iso to hyperdensity on CT and T1 iso to hyper-

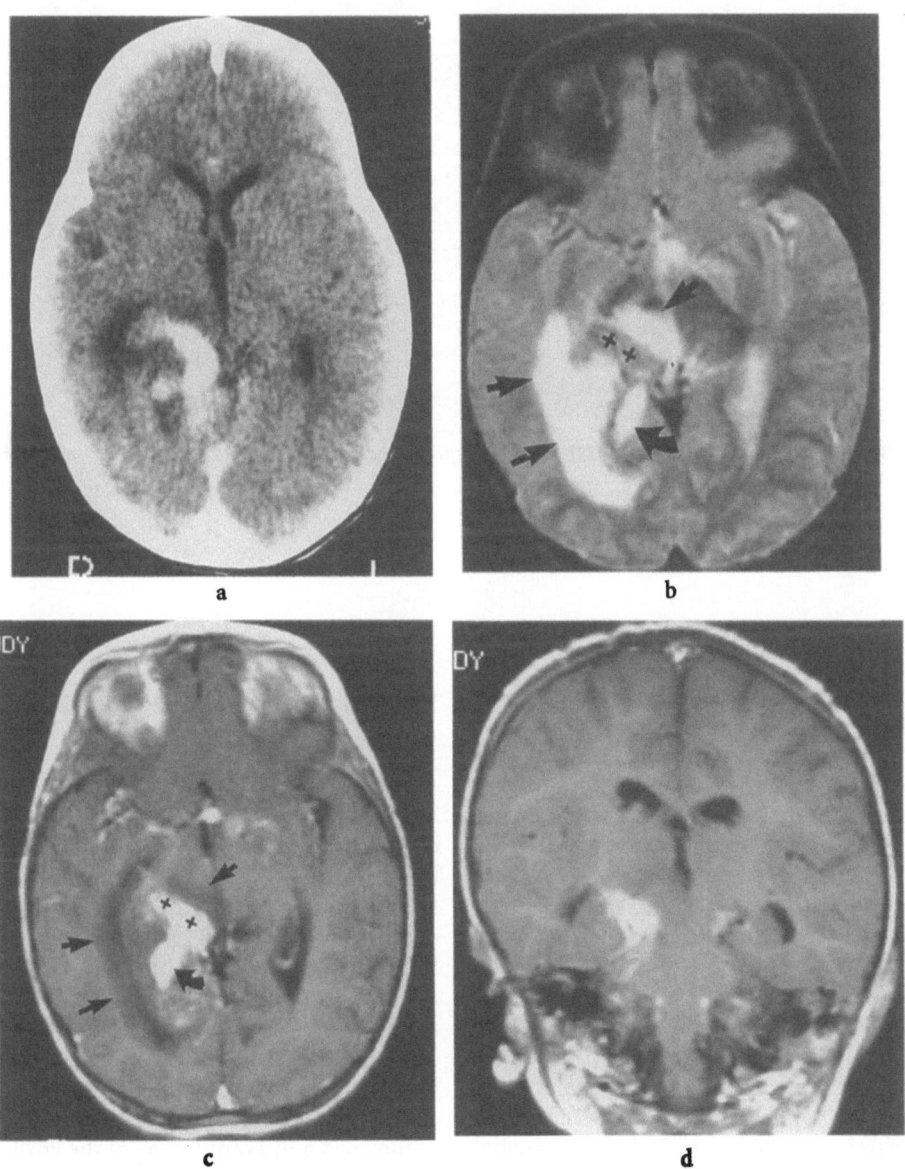

a   b

c   d

Fig. 4.25a–d. Meningeal granuloma R ambient cistern: a IV contrast-enhanced CT; enhancing granuloma with sourrounding hy-podense vasogenic edema, b axial T2 MR; granuloma (X) is largely hypointense, vasogenic edema hyperintense (straight arrows) and area of infarction hyperintense (curved arrows), c Axial IV gadolinium-enhanced T1; granuloma (X) is enhancing, vasogenic edema is not (straight arrows) but infarction does enhance (curved arrow), d coronal IV gadolinium-enhanced T1 MR: anatomic position of ambient cistern granumoma is well shown.

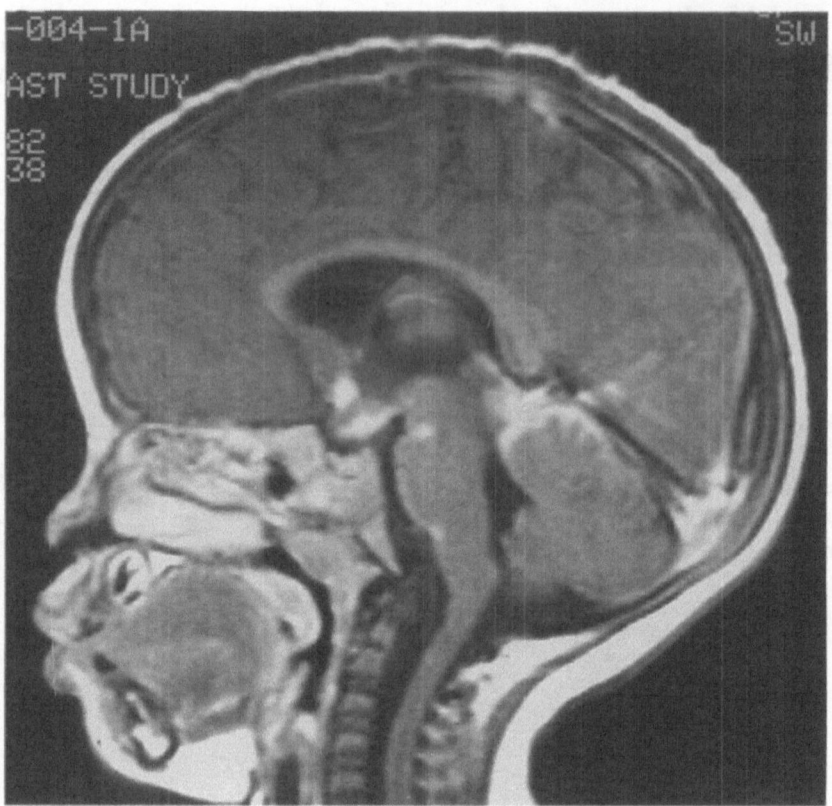

Fig. 4.26.   Sagittal IV gadolinium-enhanced T1 MR: meningeal granulomas; enhancing granulomas of the suprasellar cistern and quadrigeminal cistern demonstrated.

intensity, T2 hypointensity on MR and strong IV contrast-medium enhancement (Figs 4.25, 4.26). MR delineates the meningeal location and adjacent parenchymal involvement well. Granulomatous involvement of the meninges and superficial cortex can cause a gyral pattern of enhancement, and adjacent edema shows T1 hypointense, T2 hyperintense signal change which does not enhance on gadolinium studies. This can distinguish edema from areas of recent infarction which may enhance variably. Restriction to grey matter with little signal change evident in adjacent white matter is rarely noted (Fig. 4.27). Meningocerebral granulomas can be isolated, or present with more wide-spread meningeal disease. Appearance and progression of meningocerebral granulomas, as with parenchymal lesions, may be erratic (Figs 4.28, 4.29).

The imaging findings of intracranial tuberculoma have been reported in the literature[13,19–26].

Spinal Cord Involvement

MR is the modality of choice for visualizing spinal cord compression from subdural abscess and kyphotic deformity in TB spondylitis[27] (Ch. 6, p. 91). Long-standing bowing of the cord over a kyphotic angulation may result in cord atrophy which again MR visualizes well and non-invasively.

Focal T2 hyperintense changes in the cord itself are associated with a poor prognosis for neurological outcome[28]. This would be caused by myelopathy secondary to ischemia when vascular supply to the cord itself is compromized. Arachnoid involvement of the cord and granulomas of the cord are unusual but the use of MR evaluation will increase the detection of this pathlogy (Fig. 4.30).

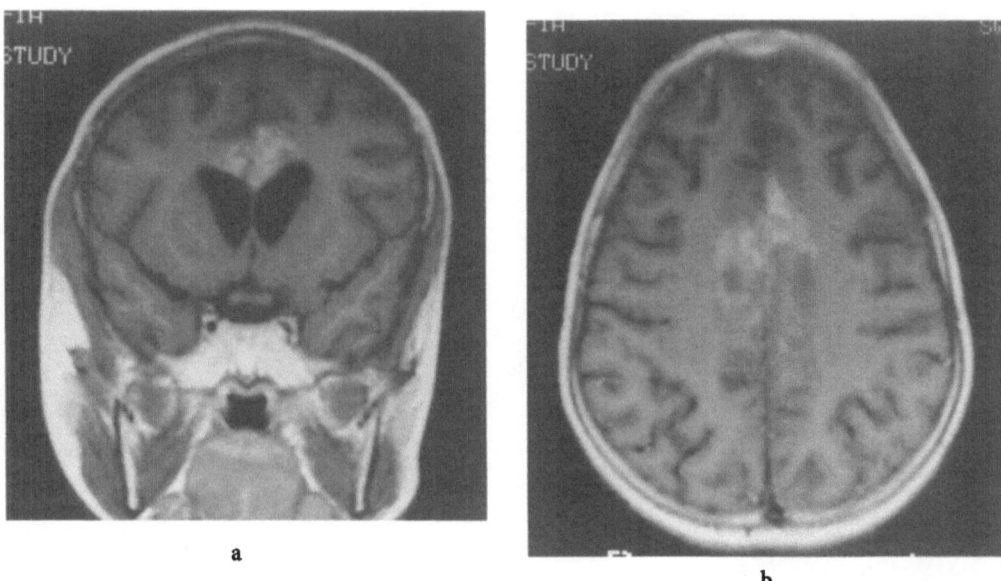

Fig. 4.27. **a** Coronal and **b** axial IV gadolinium-enhanced T1 MR: meningocerebral granulomas; meninges and adjacent grey matter enhances, note absence of basal leptomeningeal enhancement.

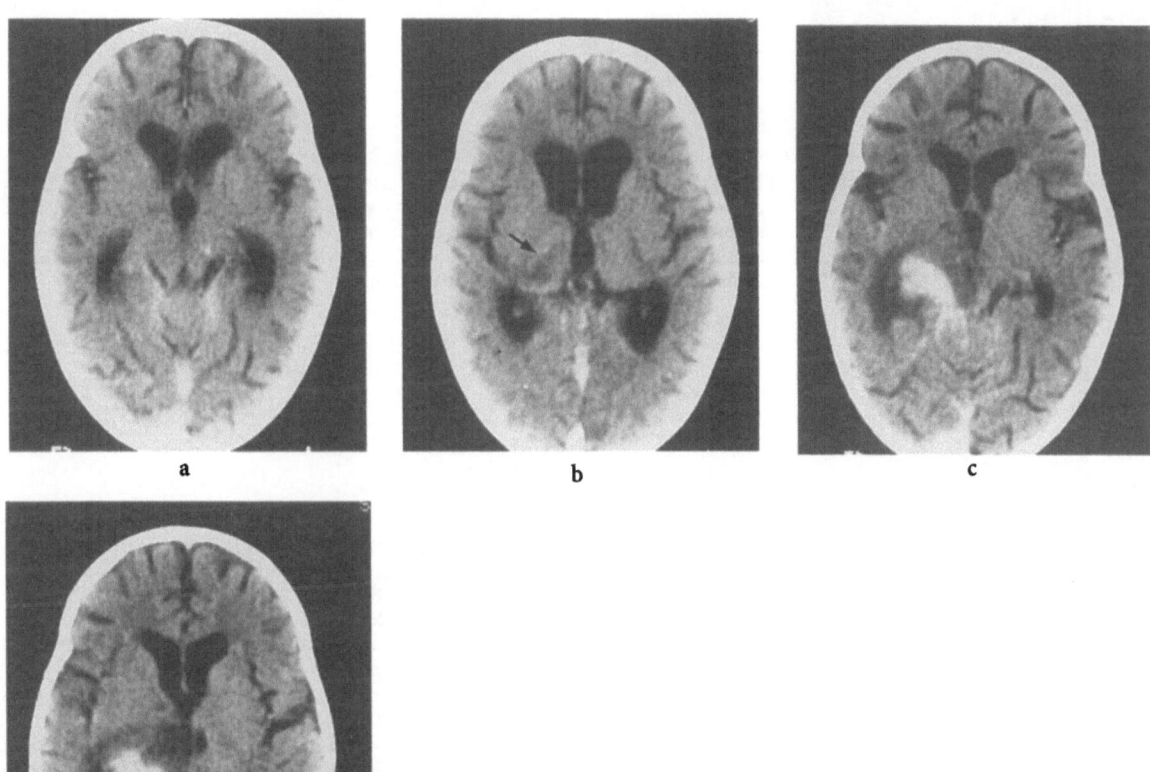

Fig. 4.28a-d. IV contrast-enhanced CT: progression of meningeal granulomas; **a,b** CT on presentation with diagnosis of tuberculous meningitis with minimal basal leptomeningeal enhancement, hydrocephalus and hypodense change of a R posterior basal ganglia infarct (arrow). **c,d** CT following 6 weeks of appropriate anti-tuberculous therapy shows persistent hydrocephalus; bilateral basal ganglia infarction is now present and a large R ambient cistern granuloma has developed with associated vasogenic edema.

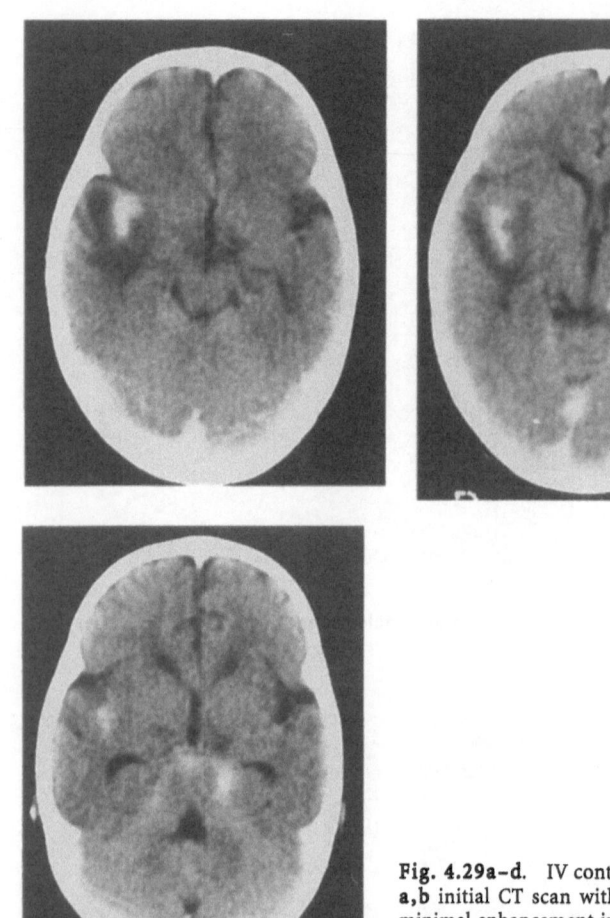
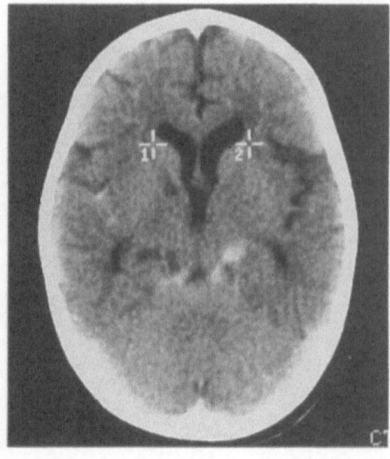

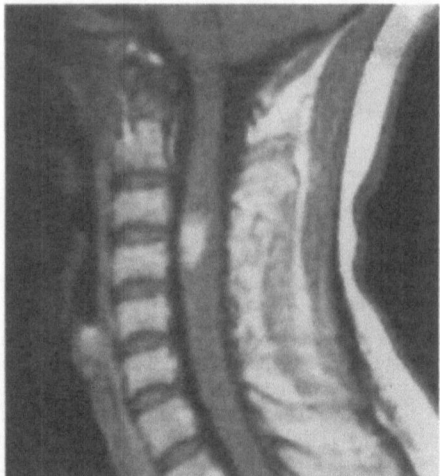

Fig. 4.29a–d. IV contrast-enhanced CT: erratic progression of meningeal granulomas; **a,b** initial CT scan with a large enhancing granuloma in the R Sylvian fissure. Note minimal enhancement in the L ambient cistern. **c,d** Scan following 3 months of anti-tuberculous therapy shows good resolution of the R Sylvian fissure granuloma but increased in enhancement of the L ambient cistern lesion.

References

1. Rich, AR, McCordock HA (1993) Pathogenesis of tuberculous meningitis. Bull Johns Hopkins Hosp. 52: 5–37
2. Kennedy DH, Fallon RJ (1979) Tuberculous meningitis. JAMA 24: 264–268
3. Medical Research Council (1948) Streptomycin treatment of tuberculous meningitis. Lancet 1: 582–596
4. Lincoln EM, Sordillo SVD, Davies PA (1960) Tuberculous meningitis in children. J Pediatr 57: 807–823
5. Donald PR, Schoeman JF, Cotton MF, Van Zyl LE (1991) Cerebrospinal fluid investigations in tuberculous meningitis. Ann Trop Pediatr 11: 241–246
6. Schoeman J, Hewlett R, Donald P (1988) MR of childhood tuberculous meningitis. Neuroradiology 30: 473–477
7. Leiguarda R, Berthier M, Starkstein S, Nogues M, Lylyk P (1988) Ischaemic infarction in 25 children with tuberculous meningitis. Stroke 19: 200–204
8. Auerbach O (1951) Tuberculous meningitis: correlation of therapeutic results with the pathogenesis and pathological changes. Am Rev Tuberc 64: 408–429

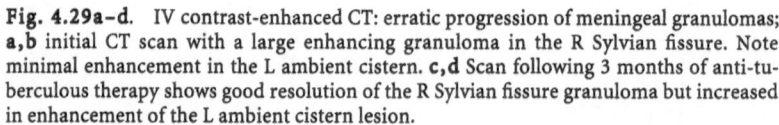

Fig. 4.30. Sagittal IV gadolinium-enhanced T1 cervical spine: enhancing tuberculoma of the cord at C4 level is demonstrated.

9. Schoeman J, Hewlett R, Donald P (1988) MR of childhood tuberculous meningitis. Neuroradiology 30: 473–477

10. Waeker NJ, Connor JD (1990) Central nervous system tuberculosis in children: a review of 30 cases. Pediatr Infect Dis J 9: 539–543

11. Mathew NT, Abraham S, Crowdy S (1973) Cerebral Angiographic features in tuberculous meningitis. Neurology 20: 1015

12. Casselman ES, Hasso AN, Ashwal S, Schneider S (1980) Computed tomography of tuberculosis meningitis in infants and children. J Cat 4: 211–216

13. Chang KH, Han MH, Roh JK, Kim IO, Han MC, Choi KS, Kim CW (1990) Gd DPTA enhanced MR imaging in intracranial tuberculosis. Neuroradiology 32: 19–25

14. Rutherfoord GS, Hewlet RH (1994) Atlas of Correlative Surgical Neuropathology and Imaging. Ch 3. Kluwer, UK

15. Rajshekar V, Haran RP, Shankar Prakash G, Chandy MJ (1993) Differentiating solitary small cysticercus granulomas and tuberculomas in patients with epilepsy. J Neurosurg 78: 402–407.

16. Domingo Z, Peter JC (1989) Intracranial tuberculomas an assessment of a therapeutic 4 drug trial in 35 children. Pediatr Neurosurg 15: 61–167

17. Peter JC, Domingo Z (1990) Response to comments on "Intracranial tuberculomas . . ." by Prakash GS et al. Pediatr Neurosurg 16: 52–53

18. Leary PM, Cremin BJ, Daubenton JD, Peter JC (1993) A study of African Children with Prolonged Focal Seizure and a specific CT Scan Finding. J Trop Pediatr 39: 176–178

19. Bhargava S, Tandon PN (1980) Intracranial tuberculomas: a CT study. BJR 53: 935–945

20. Whelan MA, Stern J (1981) Intracranial tuberculoma. Radiology 138: 75–81

21. Whelchman JM (1979) Computerized tomography of intracranial tuberculoma. Clin Rad 30: 567–573

22. Price HI, Danziger A (1978) Computer tomography in cranial tuberculosis. AJR 130: 769–771

23. Draouat S, Abdenabi B, Ghanem M, Bourjat P (1987) Computed tomography of cerebral tuberculoma. JCAT 11: 594–597

24. Gupta RK, Jena A. Sharma DK, Guha S, Khushu S, Gupta AK (1988) MR imaging of intracranial tuberculosis. JCAT 12: 280–285

25. Salgado P, Del Brutto OH, Talamas O, Zenteno MA, Rodriguez-Carbajal J (1989) Intercranial tuberculoma: MR imaging. J. Neuroradiology 31: 299–302

26. Gupta RK, Jena A, Singh AK, Sharma A, Puri V, Gupta M (1990) Role of MR in the diagnosis and management of intracranial tuberculosis. Clin Rad 41: 120–127

27. Hoffman EB, Crosier JH, Cremin BJ (1993) Imaging in Children with Spinal Tuberculosis. J Bone Joint Surg (Br) 75B: 233–239

28. Corr P, Handler L, Davey H (1991) Potts paraplegia and tuberculous spondylitis: evaluation by magnetic resonance. Neuroradiology 33(suppl): 109–110

5   Imaging of Abdominal Tuberculosis

B.J. Cremin and D.H. Jamieson

Imaging Methods

1. *Plain X-rays*
   Plain X-rays provide a non-specific preliminary examination for abdominal problems. They may be unhelpful, but may also demonstrate ascites, free gas from perforation and multiple fluid levels with dilated loops of bowel when obstruction is present. Single or multiple foci of calcification may be present in established disease.

2. *Ultrasound*
   Ultrasound is a most useful initial examination. The lack of fat in children enables the demonstration of adenopathy, bowel involvement and ascites.

3. *Barium Studies (meal and enema)*
   The use of barium meals and enemas form a good, simple and available modality to show anatomic sites of intestinal involvement, mucosal ulceration and strictures. The small bowel can be demonstrated by a follow-through examination and localized spot films, or enteroclysis may be valuable. The colon and cecum are best seen by double contrast barium enema. These studies can only infer but not demonstrate peritoneal disease.

4. *Computed Tomography (CT)*
   Computed tomography is becoming increasingly more used to evaluate acute abdominal problems. It will demonstrate adenopathy, omental and bowel involvement and ascites and has the advantage of demonstrating the full extent of abdominal involvement in one examination. Both oral and IV contrast enhancement provide optimal visualization.

5. *Magnetic Resonance Imaging (MR)*
   Magnetic resonance imaging has good potential but the costs are prohibitive for routine use and diagnostic advantages are as yet unproven[1].

Some of the largest reports of abdominal TB are from under-developed countries such as India[3,4,6,7,8,9,10] and South Africa[2,5,11,12] and concern both adults[2-5] and children[6-12]. Although gastrointestinal TB may occur without evidence of pulmonary infection on the CXR[13], the infection usually follows the ingestion of infected sputum, but hematogenous spread may be responsible for some peritoneal and organ involvement. The initial reaction of the bowel is a localized inflammation of the lymphoid tissue with subsequent necrosis. Submucosal ulcers form or there may be a hypertrophic reaction from an inflammatory fibroblastic response. A combination of both may occur. The ulcers tend to be transverse, possibly in relation to the alignment of the lymphatics[13]. Lymph node enlargement and matting together of thickened bowel and peritoneum, with subsequent fibrosis, occurs. Although the proximal colon, cecum and distal small bowel are the most common sites of involvement, the disease process may occur anywhere in the bowel.

During the 10-year period of 1980–1990, 95 children (mean age 5 years) with proven TB presented in roughly equal numbers to the medical and surgical divisions of the Red Cross Hospital at Cape Town[12]. The majority were undernourished and presented with fever, loss of weight, abdominal pain, vomiting and diarrhea. Abdominal distension (86%) and a palpable mass (57%) were the commonest physical signs and the complications that developed were obstruction (7%), abscess or fistula (7%) and perforation (4%). The overall clinical presentation of these patients was insidious, non-specific and variable. The commonest diagnostic problem was differentiating early ileo-cecal lymphoma from tuberculosis.

The disease may be divided into the three groups of adenopathy, peritoneal disease and enteric involvement. The division is artificial as these groups are not distinct[10], and there is much overlap and variability of anatomical involvement[4,12].

For purposes of description the three forms have the following imaging characteristics.

1. Adenopathy may occur without apparent gastrointestinal involvement. The enlarged nodes are seen typically in the peripancreatic, periportal, perioaortic and pericaval regions[14,15]. The mesentery and omentum may also be involved. This distribution would appear to reflect the lymphatic drainage of the involved bowel. Calcification may be seen on plain X-ray or more definitively on CT (Fig. 5.1a,b). It is flocculent in nature and does not imply that the disease process is inactive.

In children, adenopathy is best demonstrated by ultrasound. The enlarged nodes are predominantly hypoechoic with central areas that show variable acoustic echoes reflecting caseous necrosis and calcification[16,17,18]. The nodes may be discrete or matted together into large conglomerate masses (Fig. 5.2a–d). Adenopathy is also well demonstrated by CT[19-23] and typically the nodes are of low density with variable peripheral rim enhancement (Fig. 5.3a,b). There has been some histologic correlation of the non-enhancing central necrosis (caseous or liquefactive), and the enhancing inflammatory capsular and perinodal reaction[23].

2. The exudative or peritonitis form may be demonstrated both by ultrasound and CT. Three forms are described[24] and these may be distinguished by ultrasound[17].

a. "Wet" with free or loculated ascites.

b. "Dry" with caseous nodules and adhesions – "plastic peritonitis".

c. "Fibrotic-fixed" with mass formation of palpable omentum, loops of bowel or mesentery, sometimes with ascites.

The ultrasound appearance of the wet ascitic form usually is of a clear fluid which may contain multiple fixed or mobile strand-like membranes and floating debris[17]. Omental cakes and adherent small bowel loops occur. Interloop fluid between the echoic thickened bowel may give alternating echoic and echo-free bands (Fig. 5.4a) or with more matting together, a clustered appearance[18]. The fixed loops of bowel and mesentery may radiate out from the mesenteric root (Fig. 5.4b). Both the ultrasonic echo content and CT density of ascitic fluid are variable. Possibly the clear ascitic fluid represents a transudate caused by early hyperimmune

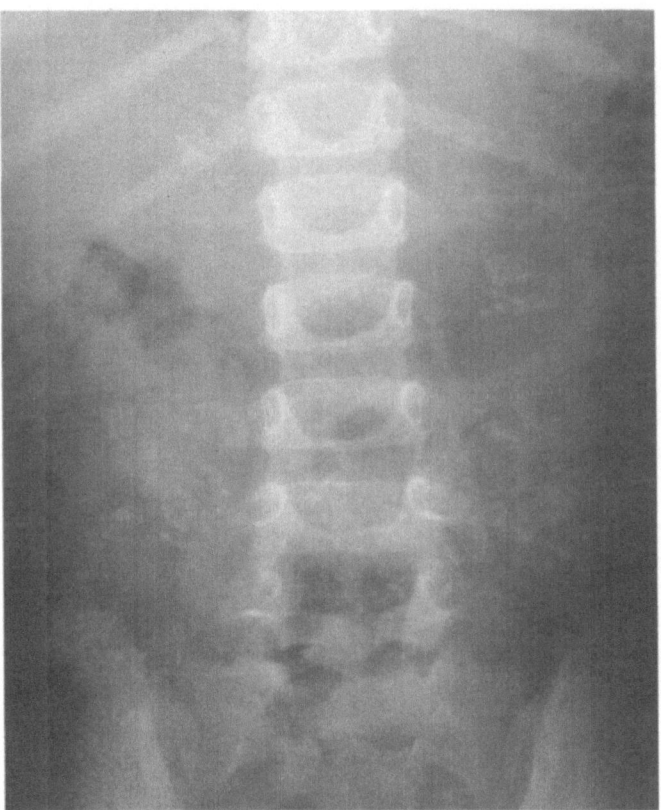

a

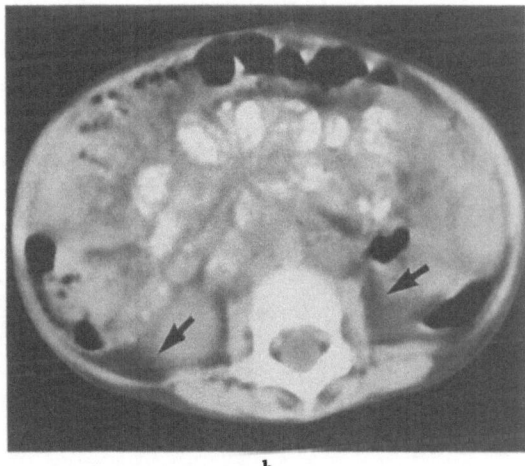

b

Fig. 5.1. a Plain X-ray, diffuse flocculent calcification. b CT, diffuse calcification of mesenteric adenopathy. There is some loculated, low density ascites (arrows).

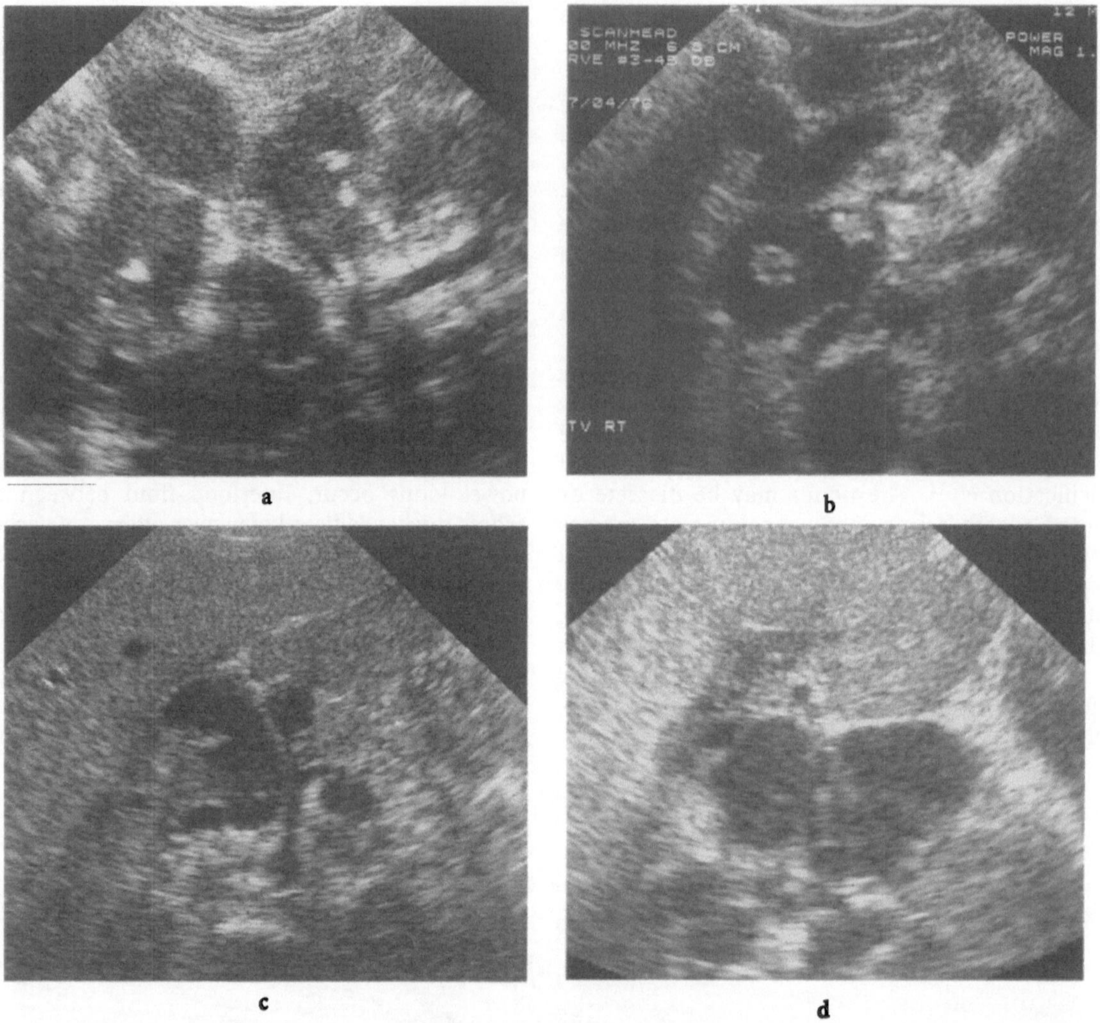

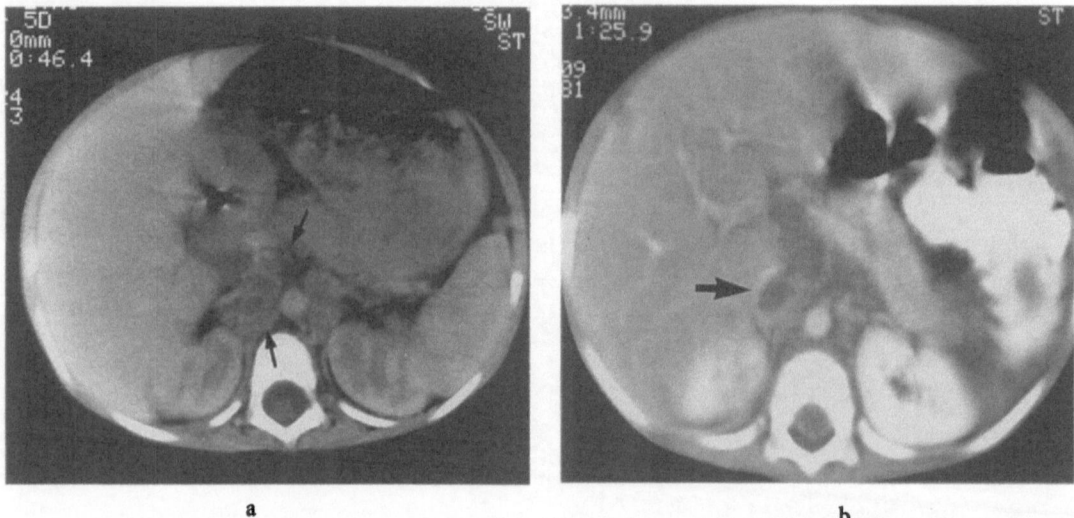

Fig. 5.2. Ultrasound. **a,b** Hypoechoic nodes containing echoic calcification in porta hepatis, **c** nodes at celiac axis, **d** at splenic hilum.

Fig. 5.3a,b. IV contrast-enhanced CT showing rim-enhancing nodes (arrows) at **a** periaortic region, **b** porta hepatis.

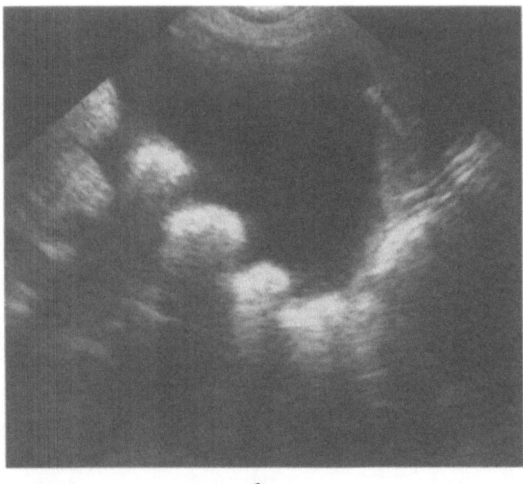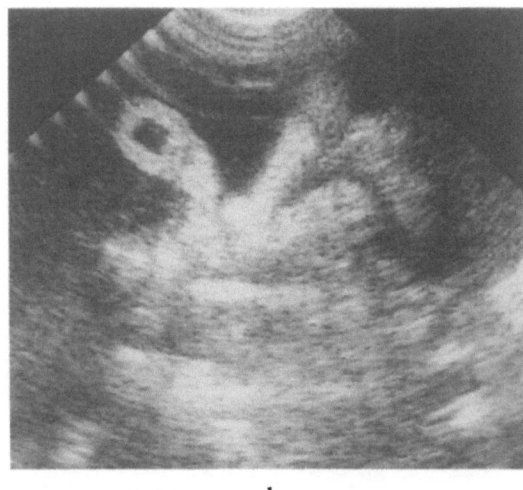

Fig. 5.4a,b. Ultrasound. **a** ascites with matted echogenic loops of bowel. **b** Ascites with echogenic bowel loops radiating from mesenteric root.

reaction and the complex fluid patterns develop later[14,17]. Cold abscesses may also be detected, as well-defined collections with thick internal echoes. These may respond to US-guided needle aspiration[18] and regress on anti-tuberculous therapy. The dry form, which may be associated with massively enlarged nodes is the commonest ultrasonic finding. When associated with adhesions they are best visualized by placing the transducer directly over the palpable masses.

CT will demonstrate ascites and omental involvement[14,19,20,21], but efficient contrast filling of the bowel is essential to differentiate thickened masses of omentum and nodes from bowel (Fig. 5.5). Dynamic IV contrast-enhanced scans will demonstrate adenopathy with low density centres and rim enhancement (Fig. 5.6a,b) that may give a multilocular appearance. The anatomic position of ascites is well shown by CT and frequently it is loculated or walled off in the abdominal cavity (Figs 5.5, 5.11, 5.12). It has been reported to be usually of relatively high density with measurements varying from 20 to 45 Hounsfield units (average of 30)[14] but there are inherent problems in using CT density measurements as absolute standards, especially when estimating small pockets of ascites.

MR after gadolinium enhancement demonstrates adenopathy (Fig. 5.7), but is an expensive alternative to simple US.

Descriptions of abdominal TB in AIDS patients have been reported in adults[25,26] and children[27,28]. When large bulky masses occur, other indolent infections, lymphoproliferative disease and metastatic Kaposi's sarcoma must be considered. It is also im-

portant to differentiate *Mycobacterium tuberculosis* (MTB) from *Mycobacterium avium intracellulare* (MAI), and in these patients fine-needle aspiration of enlarged nodes should be considered because of the difference in treatment between MTB and MAI.

3. The enteric form of the disease presents with the additional signs of abdominal pain, vomiting and ileus. In this group the plain films may be useful to demonstrate the complications of obstruction (Fig. 5.8) or perforation. The perforation may be localized and confined to a few matted loops with the resulting abscess presenting initially as an area of inflammatory edema on the bowel wall[12] or less commonly as

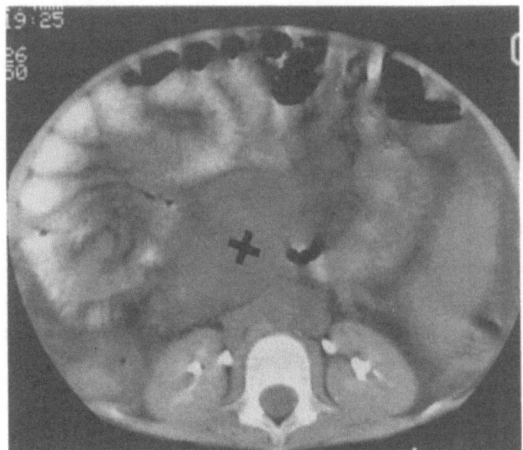

Fig. 5.5. IV contrast-enhanced CT with contrast media in bowel delineates thickened walls and separates bowel from thick omental mass (X). Loculated low density ascites is present.

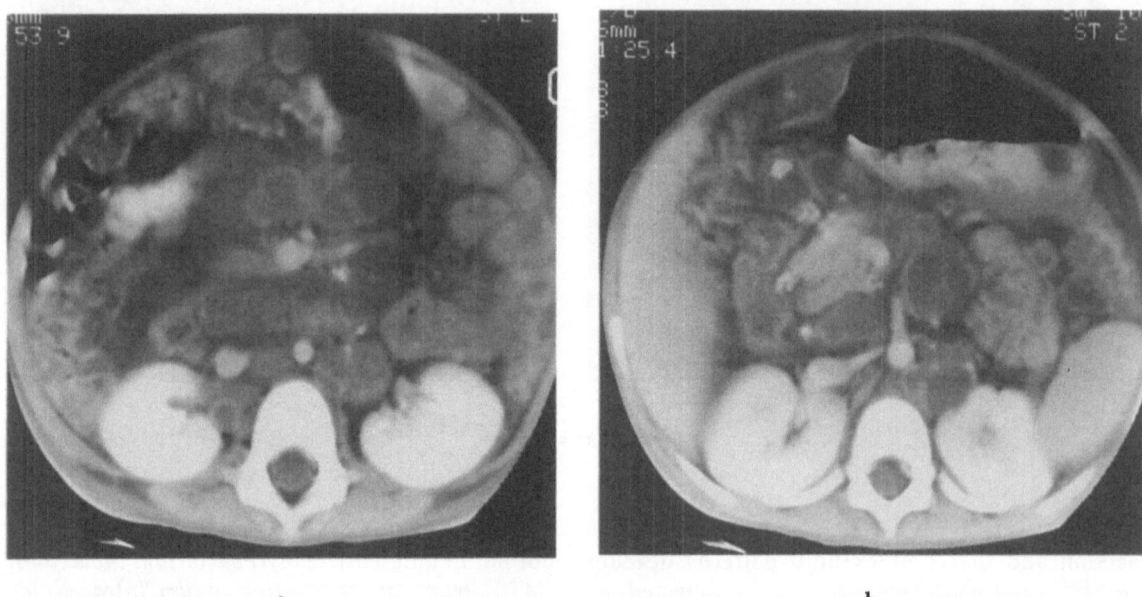

a   b

Fig. 5.6a,b.   Dynamic IV contrast-enhanced CT. **a** Multiple rim-enhancing nodes particularly in periaortic region. **b** Slice taken 1 cm caudal showing multiple nodes in right renal pelvis, omentum and beneath anterior abdominal wall.

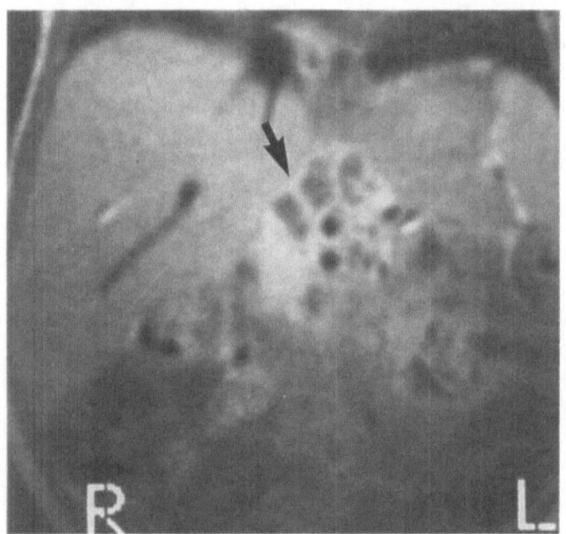

Fig. 5.7.   IV gadolinium-enhanced T1 MR showing enhancing nodal inflammatory mass (arrow) with areas of non-enhancing necrosis.

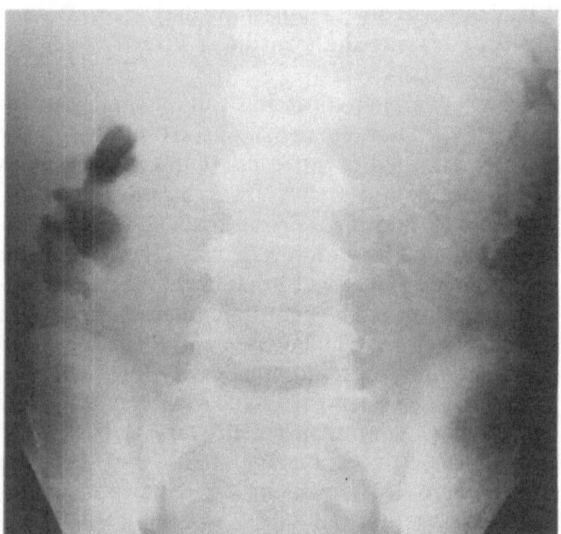

Fig. 5.8.   Plain X-ray, with faint dense diffuse calcification and a matted loop of air-containing bowel in the RIF.

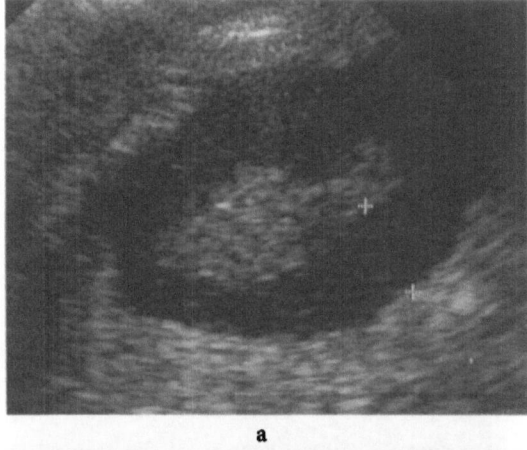

a

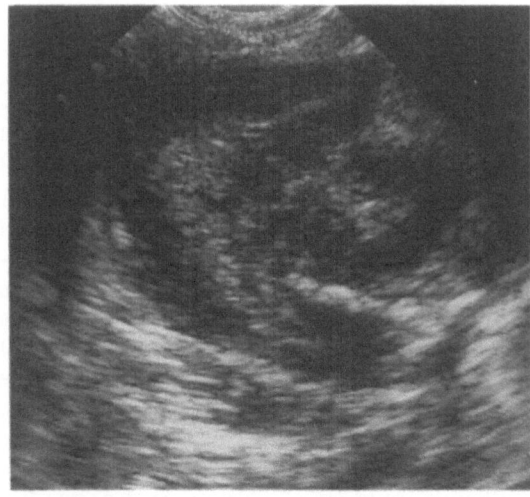

b

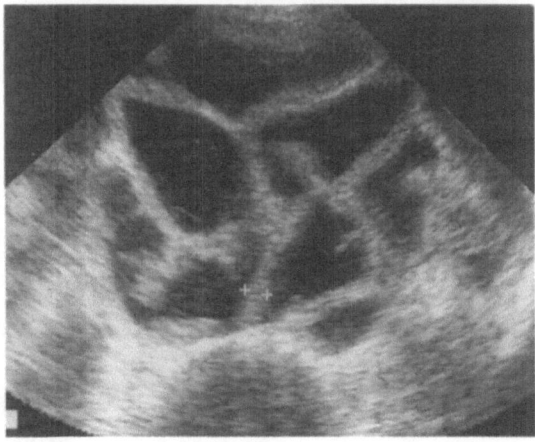

c

Fig. 5.9a–c. US series of affected bowel, a thick-walled b matted loops of thick walled bowel, c distended small bowel with echogenic walls and ascites.

a free perforation from extensive enteric involvement. Enteric cutaneous fistula formation may occur in chronic cases and require sinography.

Enteric involvement may be ulcerative, hypertrophic or combined and this may be well demonstrated by ultrasound (Fig. 5.9a,b,c). Bowel wall thickening measuring >5 mm in the small bowel when contracted and >3 mm when distended is considered pathological[29]. This is measured in transverse section from the edge of the echogenic (gas) core to the outer border of the echogenic-poor halo. Detection of an ulceration of the wall may be possible but stricture detection is poor[18]. Involvement of the ileo-cecum may cause this area to be retracted into the subhepatic region giving a pseudo-kidney sign[18] (Fig. 5.9a).

Barium studies are a simple and effective method to demonstrate enteric involvement. In the early stages of the disease, spasm and accelerated transit times are common[13]. Irregular spiculation of the bowel wall (Fig. 5.10a,b) with narrowing progressing to stricture formation occurs (Fig. 5.10c). Multiple segment disease may be seen and although there is a predilection for the ileo-cecal region, the features noted may occur anywhere in the intestinal tract. In the ileo-cecal region the ileo-cecal valve may thicken to appear as a mass in the cecum, and the whole appearance may be of fibrotic terminal ileum emptying into a rigid contracted cecum through a widely open ileo-cecal valve[13]. Involvement of the upper gastrointestinal tract is not common but involvement of the duodenum does occur and may cause bile-stained vomiting (Fig. 5.10d). Esophageal involvement with tracheobronchial fistulae is usually the result of erosion from mediastinal nodes (see Fig. 2.50).

CT also demonstrates enteric involvement after oral contrast medium (Fig. 5.11a) or IV contrast-enhancement (Fig. 5.11b). It shows the degree of bowel wall thickening and lumen narrowing, particularly in the ileo-cecal region (Fig. 5.12). The appearances include irregular thickening of the bowel wall, thickening of the ileo-cecal valve and medial wall of the cecum, with the involvement of the terminal ilium and associated adenopathy[30]. A CT diagnosis of abdominal TB may be suggested when there is high-density ascites, mesenteric thickening and enlarged lymph nodes in an appropriate clinical setting[19,21] but there are no CT findings alone or in combination that are pathognomonic of TB[14]. The facts are that none of the imaging in the modalities described is specific for tuberculosis. Abdominal malignancies such as lymphoma and inflammatory bowel disease such as Crohn's disease and other gastrointestinal infections such as giardiasis, amebiasis, yersinia, protein-losing enteropathy and intestinal malabsorbtion may mimic these features[3,6,14,19,20,22,28,30]. Attention has recently been drawn to the possibility of abdominal TB in immunosuppressed or HIV positive children[28].

The indication for surgery in cases at the Red Cross Hospital, Cape Town were[12]:

1. To gain histological diagnosis by the smallest possible laparotomy in doubtful cases.

2. Exploratory laparotomy for acute complications.

3. Definitive management of complications such as fistulae, stricture and obstruction.

Solid Organs

Granulomas of the liver and spleen are seeded by hematogenous dissemination of bacilli and are usually hypoechoic on US (Fig. 5.13a), but central echogenic areas may also be seen (Fig. 5.13b). In acute hematogenous dissemination the millet-seed-sized lesions may give a granular echoic appearance to either liver or spleen (Fig. 5.13c). They may become macronodular on US and CT[31]. In both liver and spleen, focal lesions may calcify. On CT the granulomas show focal low-density, non-enhancing areas though rim enhancement may occur[14] (Figs 5.14a,b).

Pancreatic lesions have not been reported in children. They have been reported in adults in the head of the pancreas[15] and in cases with AIDS and hematogenous dissemination[32].

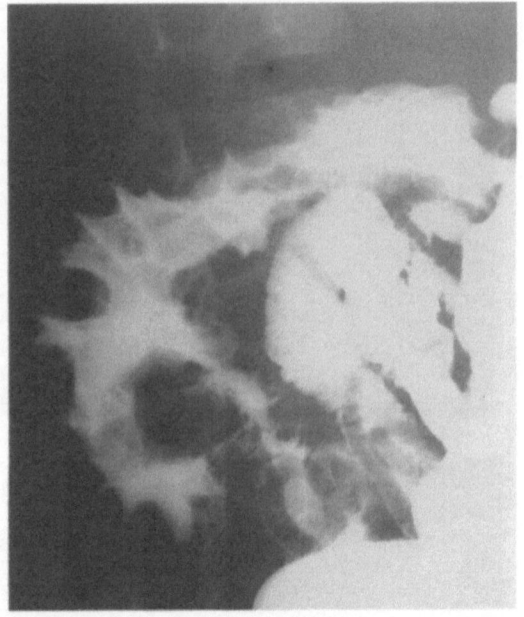

a

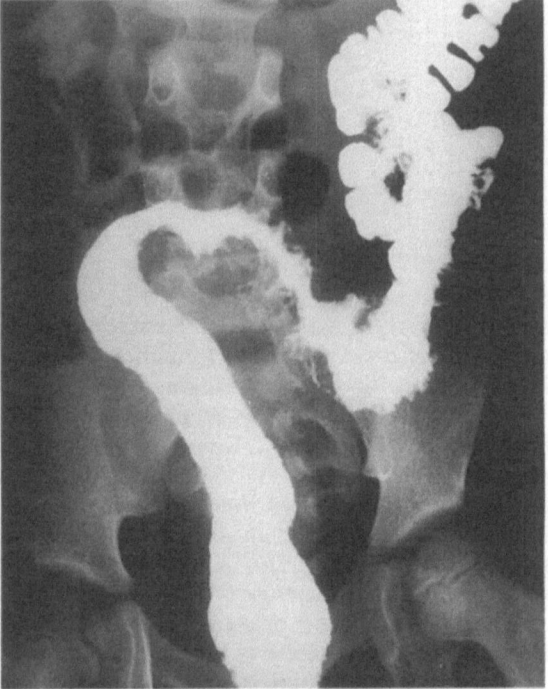

b

Fig. 5.10a–d. Barium studies. a Ileocecum with thick bowel wall showing irregular spiculations, b mucosal ulceration in sigmoid colon, c two elongated strictures in transverse colon with irregular rigid descending colon, d narrowed, irregular duodenal C loop.

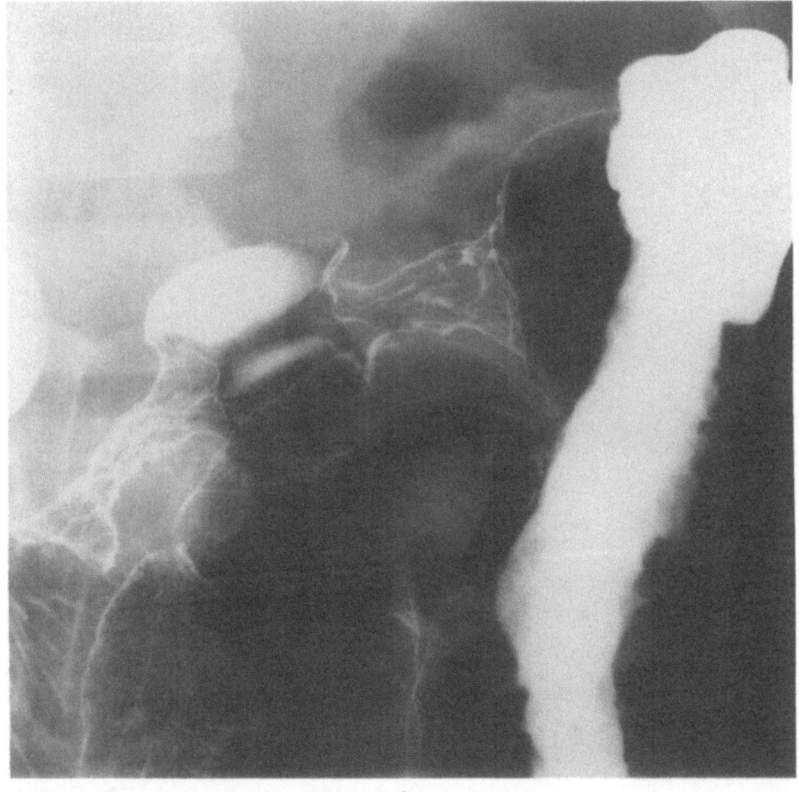

c

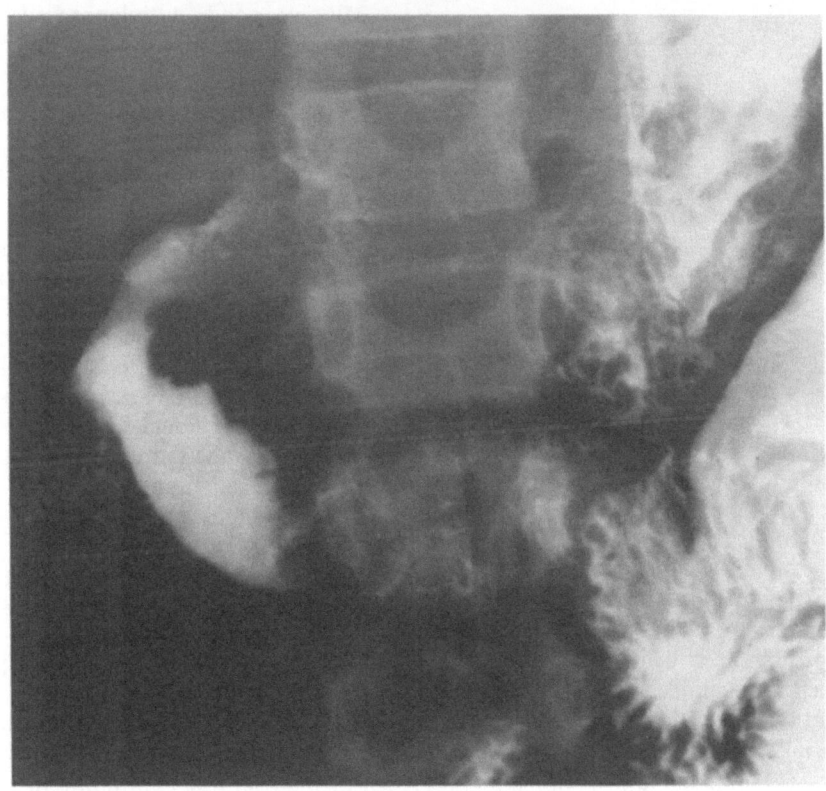

d
Fig. 5.10 (*continued*)

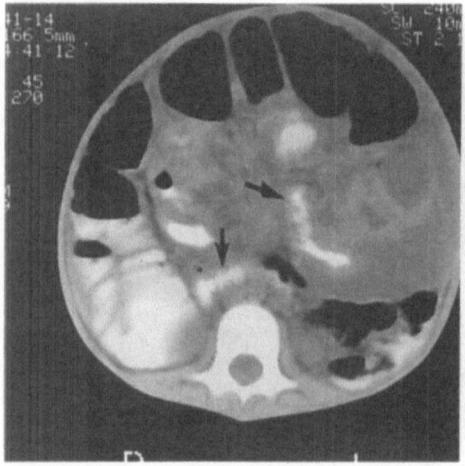
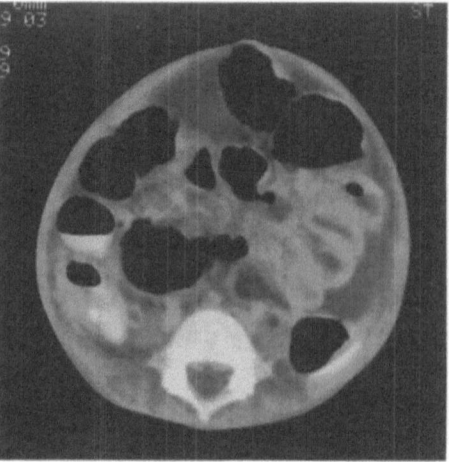

Fig. 5.11. a CT showing irregular contrast-filled ilium with mural thickening (arrows). b IV contrast – enhanced CT showing mural thickening (note similarity to US in Fig. 5.4b), low density loculated ascites is present in both studies.

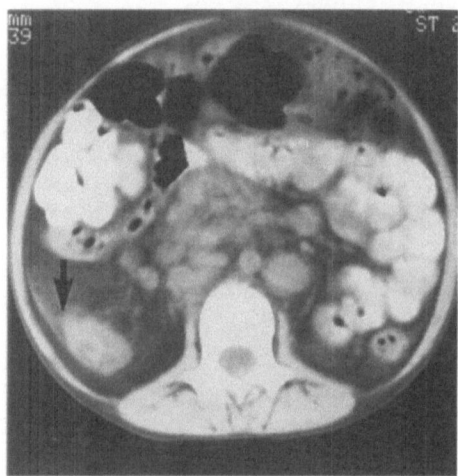

Fig. 5.12. CT showing thickened irregular contrast-filled cecum (arrow) and ascites.

Urogenital Tract

Imaging Methods

1. *Excretory Urography (EU)*
   Excretory Urography has been largely replaced by US for visualizing the kidney and bladder. It still remains an important method of visualizing the whole of the urinary tract before and after treatment. It is a relatively simple and inexpensive examination that is appreciated by clinicians.

2. *Ultrasound (US)*
   Ultrasound is non-ionizing, and is our method of choice for the initial evaluation of kidneys,

upper and lower ureters, bladder and internal genital organs.

3. *Computed Tomography (CT)*
   Computed tomography gives good visualization of renal pathology and after contrast enhancement provides some information on renal function.

4. *Magnetic Resonance Imaging (MR)*
   MR gives good multiplanar visualization but has no real diagnostic advantage over EU and CT.

5. *Radioisotopes*
   DMSA and MAG3 studies are recommended for estimating renal parenchyma and function, which is important if any surgical treatment is envisaged.

Renal tuberculosis is a silent disease seen more commonly in adults[33-36] than in children[37-39]. A long latent period between the initial infection and urogenital manifestation is characteristic. An interval of 36 years between initial childhood bone infection and adult epididymitis has been recorded[36]. In children our usual incidence is at the end of the first decade[39] and although infection is bilateral, the presentation is usually unilateral.

The bacilli involve the kidneys via hematogenous spread and the tuberculous foci may heal, lie dormant or spread into the collection system to involve the renal pyramids[40]. The parenchymal focus ulcerates and ruptures into the calyx, causing cavitation and calyceal irregularities. This progresses to large multiple cavities with destruction of renal parenchyma in which the caseating material may calcify to create a speckled or amorphous appearance. Strictures commonly occur at points of narrowing such as the infundibulum, ureter–pelvic

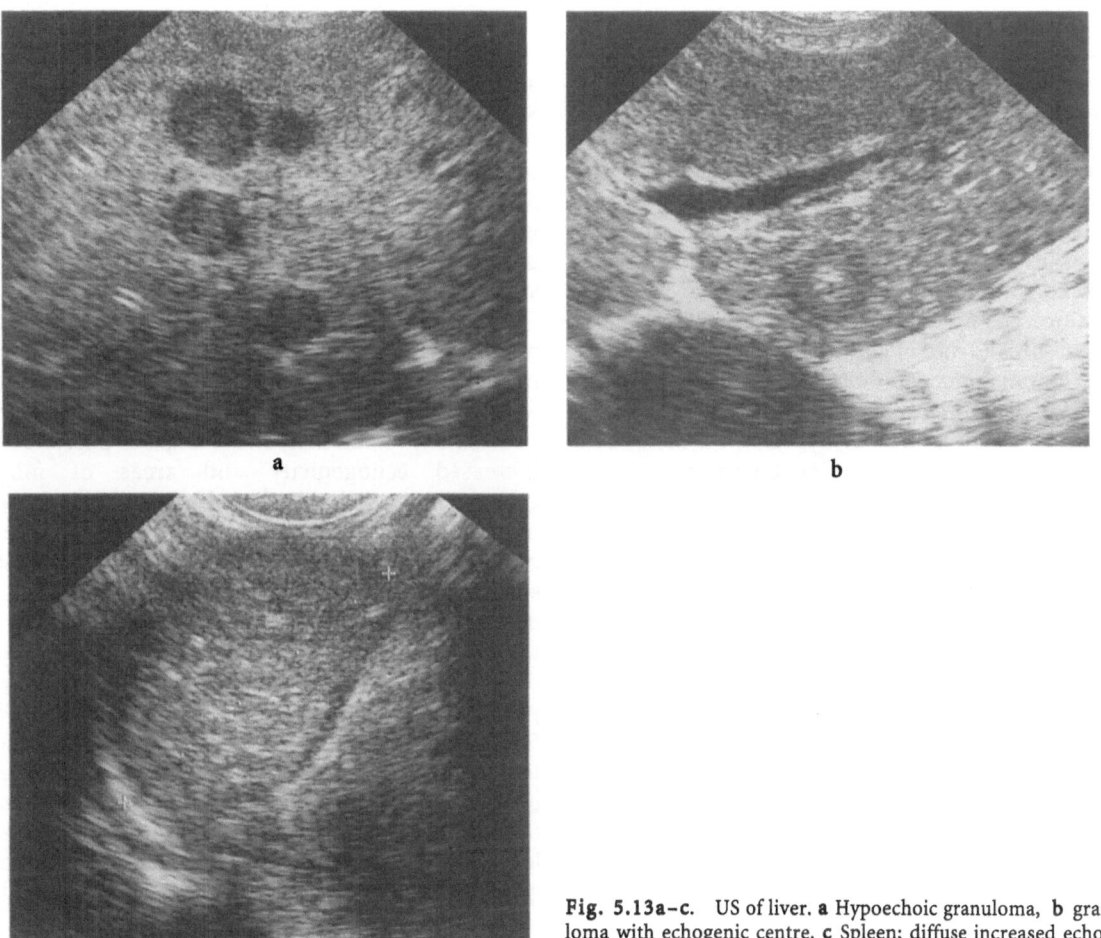

Fig. 5.13a–c. US of liver. **a** Hypoechoic granuloma, **b** granuloma with echogenic centre. **c** Spleen; diffuse increased echogenicity due to small wide-spread focal granulomas.

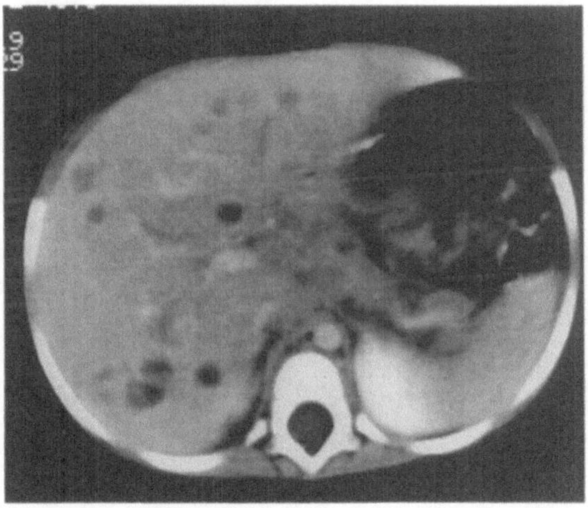

Fig. 5.14a,b. IV contrast-enhanced CT showing, **a** non-enhancing granulomas of liver, **b** in liver (arrow) and spleen. Adenopathy is present at splenic hilum (curved arrow).

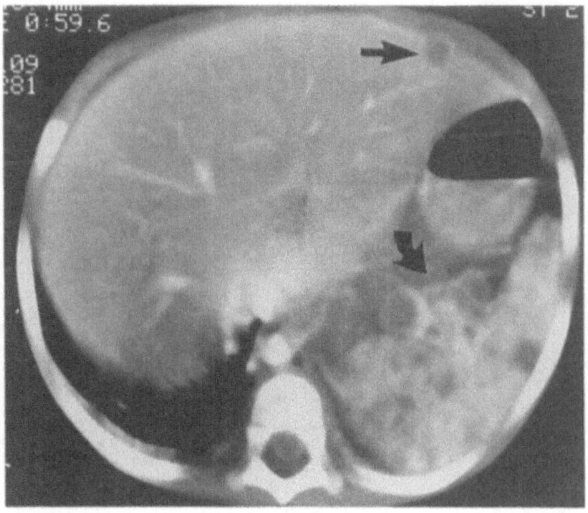

junction and distal ureter. When the entire collecting system is obstructed, autonephrectomy ensues and this is a common occurrence when presentation is delayed in children[39-41]. Ureters develop uroepithelial granulomas which are irregular and progress to fibrosis with strictures and proximal dilation to give them a beaded or pipe-stem configuration.

Bladder involvement is a progression of uroepithelial involvement and results in fibrosis and irregular constrictions which distort the vesico-ureteric junction causing reflux or obstruction. Tuberculous epidydimitis is rare in children; it may be secondary to retrograde infection, but direct hematogenous infection is the more usual mode of infection[34].

The clinical features of dysuria, frequency and hematuria may not be prominent, even in advanced disease. The occurrence of a sterile pyuria, microscopic hematuria and an acid urinary pH are strong indicators of tuberculosis infection, and skin testing is usually positive. Urine culture may give positive information in 50%[39] to 80% of cases[36]. In suspected cases, a minimum of 6 early morning urine specimens should be sent for culture.

The imaging of tuberculous pathology is well seen by excretory urography. The early calyceal destruction and cavitation may be demonstrated (Fig. 5.15a,b). Small cavities fill by dependant drainage and may not be visible on early films. Hydronephrosis, secondary to stricture, and obstruction of the collecting system may occur (Fig. 5.16) and cause further damage to renal tissues. However, the "hydronephrotic" appearance may also result from destructive cavitation within the kidney. A non-functioning kidney or autonephrectomy is the end stage of the disease and was found in half our patients on presentation[41] (Fig. 5.16b, 5.17). Excretory urography is also the best modality to demonstrate the entire length of the ureters for assessing irregularity and sites of strictures.

Ultrasound also provides a highly accurate assessment of urogenital tuberculosis[41-44]. Identification of irregular and dilated calyces and cavities correlates well with excretory urography findings (Fig. 5.18). Assessment of parenchymal changes is possible and increased echogenicity and areas of mixed echogenicity surround calyceal lesions[41]. Focal granulomatous lesions may be identified. Echoic calcification may be dense enough to cast acoustic shadows. Hydronephrosis, whether obstructive or destructive, is well visualized and echoic debris in the collecting systems is invariably noted. Late-stage disease may show an intensely echogenic small renal pelvis caused by fibrosis and cicatrization (Fig. 5.19). Dilated ureters can be demonstrated in their upper (Fig. 5.18c) and lower regions (Fig. 5.20a) and bladder involvement is well shown. Echogenic uroepithelial irregularity and granulomatous mass lesions are well seen in the full bladder. The progression to a thick-walled, small-volume bladder

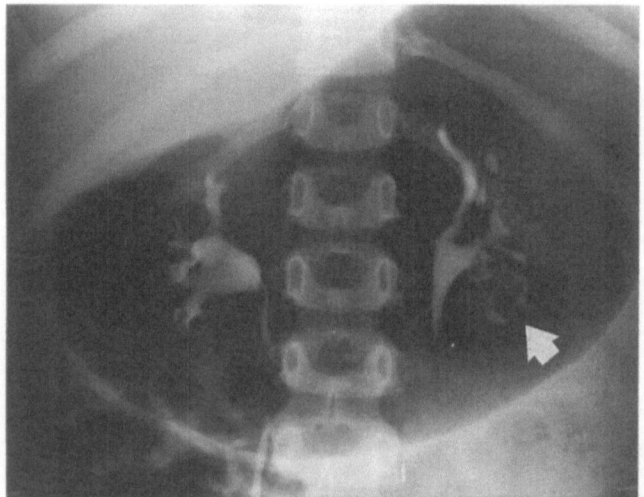

a

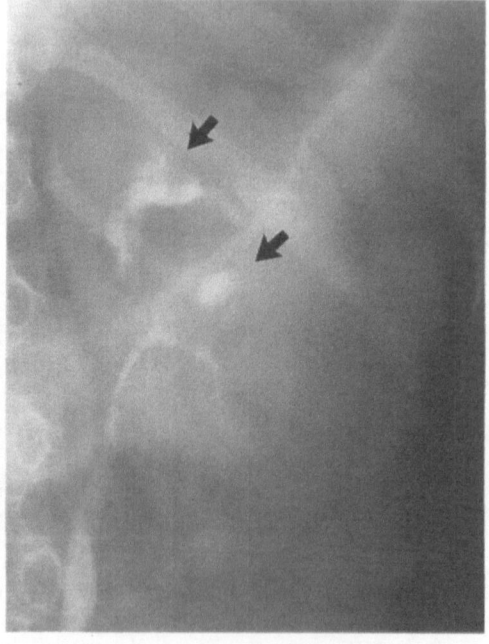

b

Fig. 5.15a,b. Excretory urography. **a** destruction of lower calyces in the left kidney with formation of crescents as contrast media outlines the cavity edges (arrow). **b** destruction of upper and middle calyces with cavity formation (arrows). It is typical that cavities fill late by dependant drainage from the affected calyces.

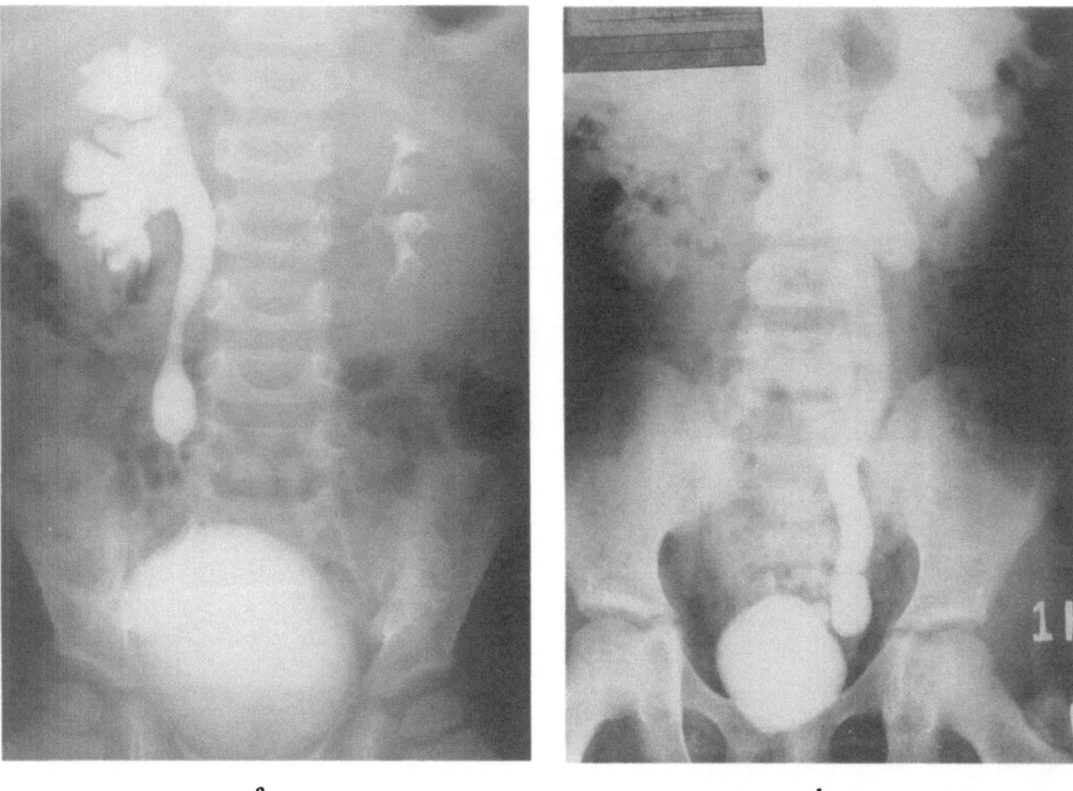

a   b

Fig. 5.16a,b. Excretory urography. **a** Hydronephrosis of right kidney due to stricture of distal ureter. **b** Delayed 1-h film showing hydronephrosis of left kidney with small contracted bladder and distal ureter stricture. The right kidney has an autonephrectomy with some diffuse calcification.

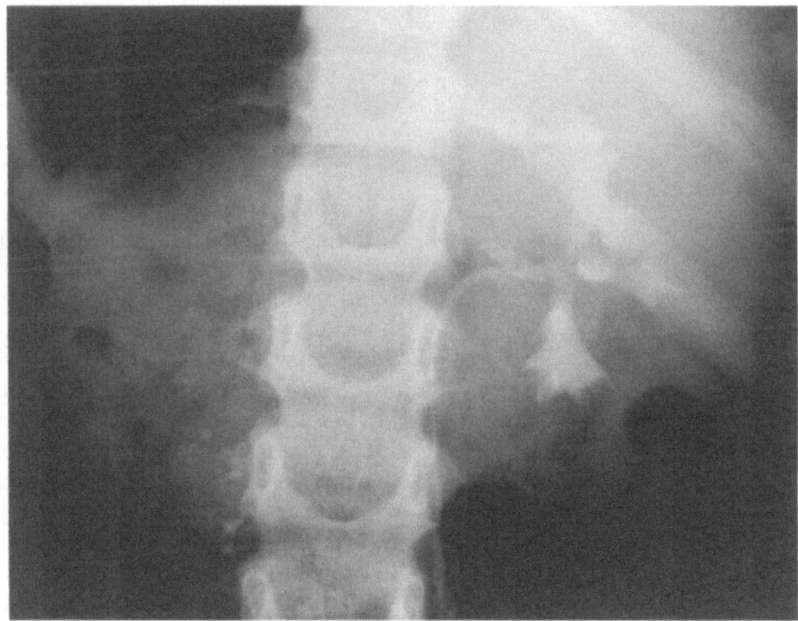

Fig. 5.17. Excretory urography. Autonephrectomy of right kidney with speckled calcification.

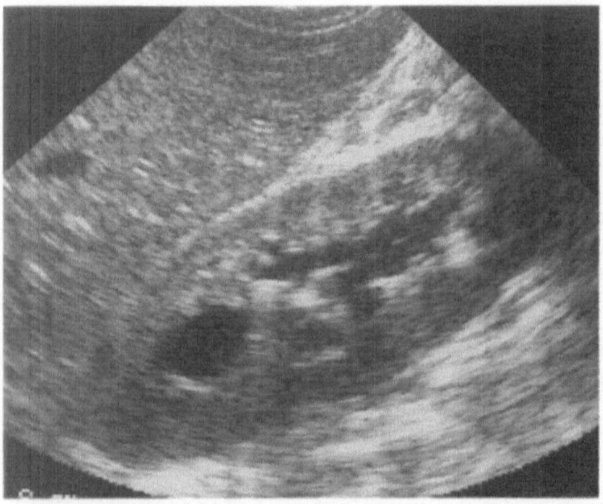

Fig. 5.18a–c. Ultrasound. a,b demonstrating irregular caliectasis with echogenic foci in parenchyma, c irregular cavitation with dilation of upper ureter and uroepithelial thickening.

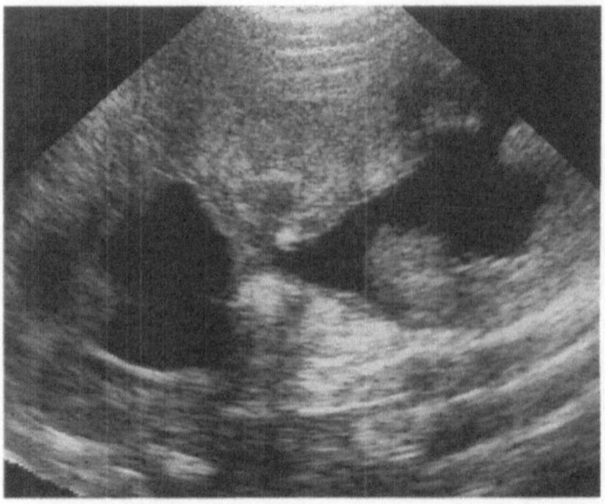

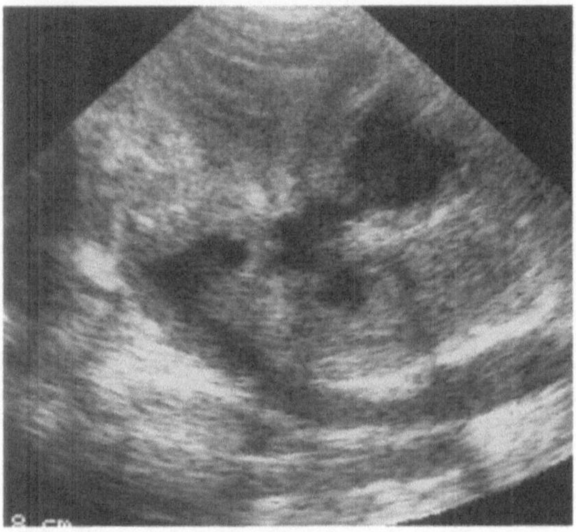

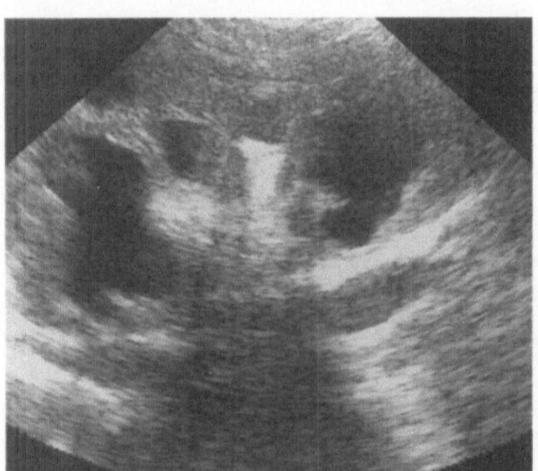

Fig. 5.19. Ultrasound of autonephrectomized kidney with echogenic material blocking the renal pelvis.

with gaping ureteric orifices may be visualized (Fig. 5.20b,c).

Computed tomography provides excellent cross-sectional anatomy of renal (Fig. 5.21) and bladder pathology (Fig. 5.22a,b). Its superiority over ultrasound in this regard must be balanced against cost and availability. MR provides multiplanar imaging (Fig. 5.23) without ionization but no clear diagnostic advantage over more conventional imaging modalities. Radio-isotope studies including MAG3 and DSMA provide excellent information about renal function in residual renal parenchyma and are helpful in assessing prognosis.

The overall imaging appearances as described are fairly specific for urinary tract tuberculosis, but conditions such as xanthogranulomatous pyelonephritis[45] may give similar appearances, particularly on ultrasound examination. In the kidney, conditions

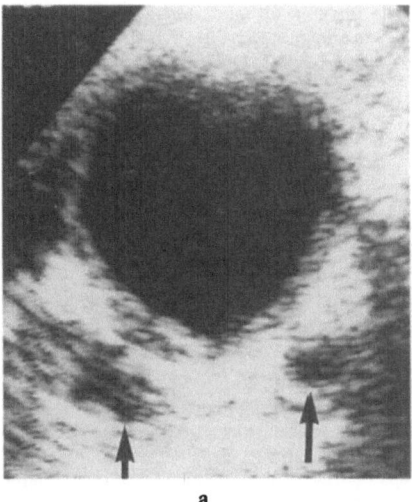

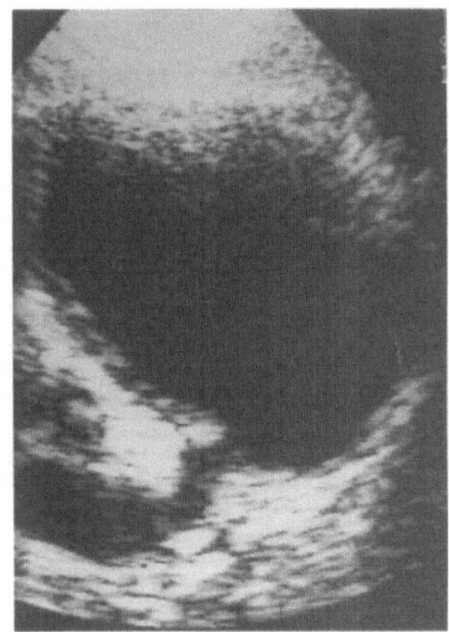

Fig. 5.20a,b. Ultrasound, showing irregular contracted bladder with dilated ureters in **a** transverse (arrows) and **b** sagittal projections.

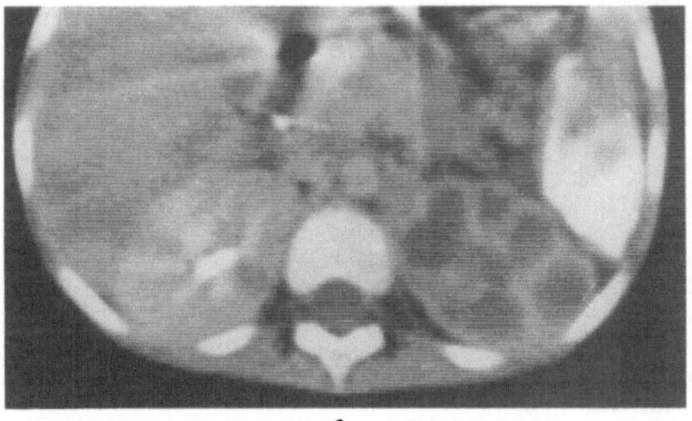

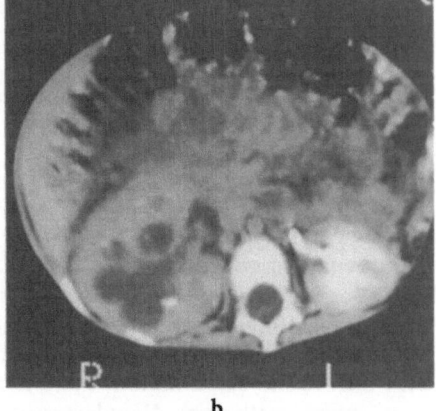

Fig. 5.21a,b. Contrast CT showing **a** L autonephrectomized kidney, **b** irregular destruction of calyceal system in R kidney.

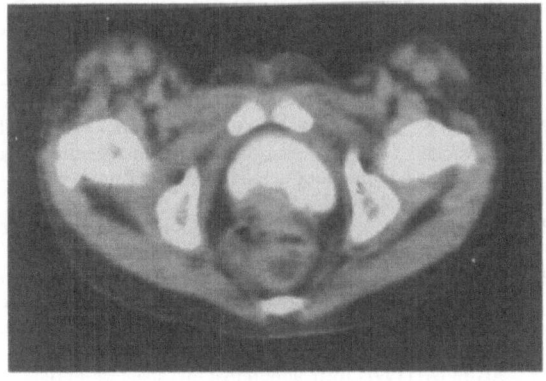

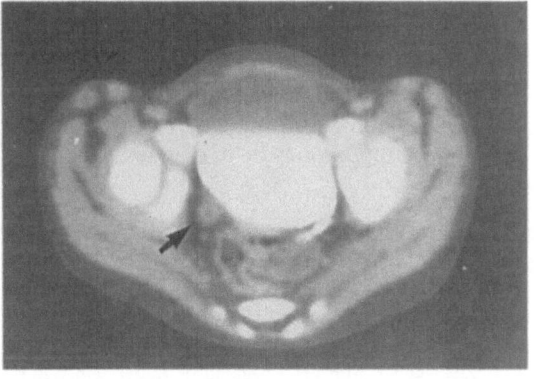

Fig. 5.22a. Contrast-enhanced CT showing involvement of bladder base. **b** R distal ureter and adjacent bladder (arrow).

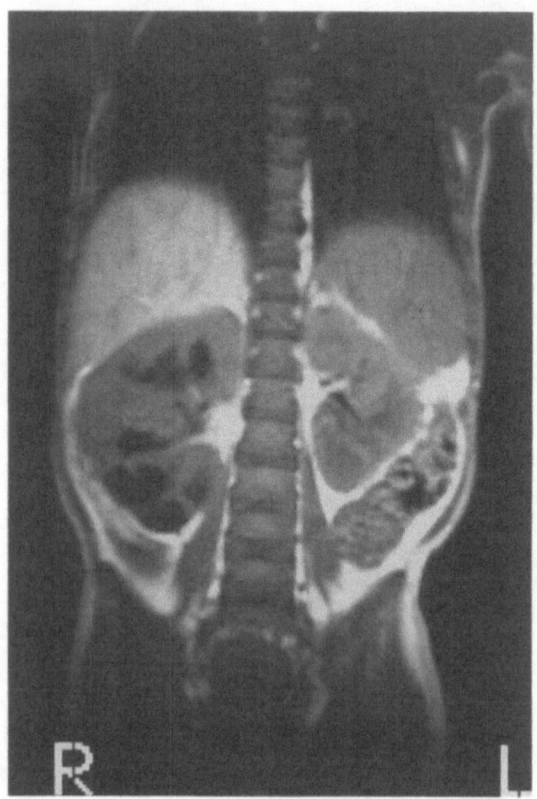

Fig. 5.23. Coronal T1 MR demonstrating irregular cavitation in left kidney (same case as shown in Fig. 5.21b).

causing papillary necrosis, such as sickle cell disease and phenacatin overdose, have to be excluded and calyceal diverticula may also be considered. The latter are smooth-walled, occurring predominantly in the upper group of calyces and, when correlated with ultrasound examination, there is no adjacent parenchymal pathology. Neoplasms of the bladder and, in endemic regions, granulomatous conditions such as bilharzia may have to be considered in the differential diagnosis.

If diagnostic confirmation of tuberculosis is not obtained from urinary samples, or associated clinical criteria, then bladder biopsy, retrograde ureter catheter sampling and imaging-directed needle aspiration for biopsy may be of diagnostic value.

References

1. Zirinsky KZ, Auh YH, Kneeland JB, Ruberstein WA, Kazam E (1985) Computed tomography, sonography, and MR imaging of abdominal tuberculosis. J Comput Assist Tomogr 9: 961–963
2. Werbeloff L, Novis BH, Bank S, Marks IN (1973) Radiology of tuberculosis of the gastrointestinal tract. Br J Radiol 46: 329–336
3. Das P, Shukla HS (1976) Clinical diagnosis of abdominal tuberculosis. Br J Surg 63: 941–946
4. Bhansali SK (1977) Abdominal tuberculosis. Experiences with 300 cases. Am J Gastroenterol 67: 324–337
5. Gilinsky NH, Marks IN, Kottler RE, Price SK (1983) Abdominal tuberculosis. A 10-year review. S Afr Med J 64: 849–857
6. Mitra SK, Yadav K, Mehta S, Kumar L, Pathak IC (1978) Abdominal tuberculosis in children. Indian J Surg 40: 96–100
7. Madhok P, Kapur VK (1982) Abdominal tuberculosis in children. Prog Pediatr Surg 15: 173–180
8. Chavalittamrong B, Talalak P (1982) Tuberculous peritonitis in children. Prog Pediatr Surg 15: 161–167
9. Dwiwedi BD (1982) Abdominal tuberculosis in children. Prog Pediatr Surg 15: 169–171
10. Nagi B, Duggal R, Gupta R, Mehta S (1987) Tuberculous peritonitis in children. Pediatr Radiol 17: 282–284
11. Johnson CAC, Hill ID, Bowie MD (1987) Abdominal tuberculosis in children. A survey of cases at the Red Cross War Memorial Children's Hospital, 1976–1985. S Afr Med J 72: 20–22
12. Millar AJW, Rode H, Cywes S (1990) Abdominal tuberculosis in children – surgical management. Pediatr Surg Int 5: 392–396
13. Thoeni RF, Margulis AR (1979) Gastrointestinal tuberculosis. Semin Roentgenol 14: 283–294
14. Hulnick DH, Megibow AJ, Naidich DP, Hilton S, Cho KC, Balthazar EJ (1985) Abdominal tuberculosis: CT evaluation. Radiology 157: 199–204
15. Denton T, Hossain J (1993) A radiological study of abdominal tuberculosis in a Saudi population, with special reference to ultrasound and computed tomography. Clin Radiol 47: 409–414
16. Ozkan K, Gurses N, Gurses N (1987) Ultrasound appearance of tuberculous peritonitis. J Clin Ultrasound 15: 350–352
17. Lee DH, Lim JH, Ko YT, Yoon Y (1991) Sonographic findings in tuberculous peritonitis of wet-ascitis type. Clin Radiol 44: 306–310
18. Kedar RP, Shah PP, Shivde RS, Malde HM (1994) Sonographic findings in gastrointestinal and peritoneal tuberculosis. Clin Radiol 49: 24–29
19. Epstein BM, Mann JH (1982) CT of abdominal tuberculosis. AJR 139: 861–866
20. Hanson RD, Hunter TB (1985) Tuberculous peritonitis: CT appearance. AJR 144: 931–932
21. Dahlene DH, Stanley RJ, Koehler RE, Shin MS, Tishler JMA (1984) Abdominal tuberculosis: CT findings. J Comput Assist Tomogr 8: 443–445
22. Denath FM (1990) Abdominal tuberculosis in children: CT findings. Gastrointest Radiol 15: 303–306
23. Pombo F, Rodriquez E, Mato J, Pere-Fontan J, Rivera E, Valvuena L (1992) Patterns of contrast enhancement of tuberculous lymph nodes demonstrated by computed tomography. Clin Radiol 46: 13–17
24. Stassa G (1967) Tuberculous peritonitis. Am J Roentgen 101: 409–413
25. Perich J, Ayuso MC, Vilana R, Ayuso JR Cardenal, Mallofré C (1990) Disseminated lymphatic tuberculosis in acquired immuno deficiency syndrome: computed tomographic findings. Can Assoc Radiol J 51: 353–357
26. Radin DR (1991) Intra abdominal mycobacterium tuberculosis vs mycobacterium avium-intracellulare infection in

patients with AIDS distrinction based on CT findings. AJR 156: 487–491

27. Haller JO, Cohen HL (1994) Gastrointestinal manifestations of Aids in children. AJR 162: 387–393

28. Ablin DS, Jain KA, Azouz Em (1994) Abdominal tuberculosis in children. Pediatr Radiol 24: 473–477.

29. Bluth EI, Merritt CRB, Sullivan MA (1979) Ultrasonic evaluation of the stomach, small bowel and colon. Radiology 133: 677–680

30. Balthazar EJ, Gordon R, Hulnick D (1990) Ileocecal tuberculosis: CT and radiologic evaluation. AJR 154: 499–503

31. Levine C (1990) Primary macro nodular hepatic tuberculosis. US and CT appearances. Gastrointest Radiol 15: 307–309

32. Levine R, Scott T, Steinberg W, Ginsberg A, Brown M, Huntington D (1992) Tuberculous abscess of the pancreas. Case report and review of the literature. Dig Dissci 377: 1141–1144

33. Roylance J, Penry JB, Davis ER, Roberts M (1970) The radiology of tuberculosis of the urinary tract. Clin Radiol 21: 163–170

34. Gow JG (1971) Genito urinary tuberculosis. A study of the disease in one unit over a period of 24 years. Ann R Coll Surg Engl ; 49: 52–69

35. Kollins SA, Hartman GW, Carr DT, Segura JW, Hattery RA (1974) Roentgenographic findings in urinary tract tuberculosis. A 10 year review. AJR 121: 487–498

36. Christensen WI (1974) Genitourinary tuberculosis: Review of cases. Medicine 53: 377–390

37. Lattimer JK, Boyes T (1958) Renal tuberculosis in children. Pediatrics 22: 1193–1200

38. Ehrich RM, Lattimer JK (1971) Urogenital tuberculosis in children. J Urology 105: 461–465

39. Aaronson IA (1987) Urogenital tuberculosis in children. S Afr Med J 71: 424–426

40. Tonkin AK, Witten DM (1979) Genitourinary tuberculosis. Semin Roentgenol 24: 305–318

41. Cremin BJ (1987) Radiological imaging of urogenital tuberculosis in children with emphasis on ultrasound. Pediatr Radiol 17: 34–38

42. Schaffer R, Becker JA, Goodman J (1983) Sonography of tuberculous kidney. Urology 22: 209–211

43. Premkumar A, Lattimer J, Newhouse JH (1987) CT and sonography of advanced urinary tract tuberculosis. AJR 148: 65–69

44. Das KM, Indudhara R, Vaidyanathan S (1991) Sonographic featues of genitourinary tuberculosis. AJR 158: 327–329

45. Cousins C, Somers J, Broderick N, Rance C, Shaw D (1994) Xantho-granulomatous pyelonephritis in childhood: ultrasound and CT diagnosis. Pediatr Radiol 24: 210–212

6 Imaging of Skeletal Tuberculosis

B.J. Cremin and D.H. Jamieson

Imaging Methods

1. *Plain X-rays*
   This is the major imaging modality for skeletal disease. Lateral tomography is useful for evaluating spinal lesions.
2. *Computed Tomography (CT)*
   CT is not usually essential for non-spinal disease. In the spine, CT demonstrates not only early disease but also involvement of the posterior elements and spinal canal encroachment.
3. *Magnetic Resonance Imaging (MR)*
   Magnetic resonance imaging is the best modality to demonstrate spinal disease for the extent of abscess formation and cord compression. It may be helpful in differentiating other conditions and may also show further unexpected early skeletal lesions. Gadolinium studies demonstrate rim enhancement of TB abscesses.
4. *Ultrasound (US)*
   Ultrasound may be used to show the extent of a paraspinal mass but this is best demonstrated by CT or MR.
5. *Isotopes*
   Isotopes can be used to show the extent and distribution of multiple lesions. Pin-hole collimators and single photon emission tomography (SPECT) increase the spatial resolution but the results are non-specific.

Three general points about skeletal TB in young children should be emphasized.

1. The disease commences as an indolent (painless) non-acute lesion. There are exceptions, but in the early stages pain is not a prominent feature. It occurs later and is a warning sign of the mechanical effects of joint involvement or abscess formation.
2. The osteoarticular lesions affect predominantly the weight-bearing joints and may be initially exudative. This involvement of synovia may be either direct or from adjacent infection, and is eventually the cause of cartilage destruction and joint space narrowing. The early appearances of osteoarticular infection may be hyperemic and cause osteopenia before destructive bone and joint changes occur.
3. In growing bones the osseous lesion is usually metaphyseal. It is both destructive and proliferative and causes a lytic and expansile lesion with a "cystic" appearance. The term cystic is preferred to "pseudocystic". It does not imply fluid-containing.

Although skeletal tuberculosis is predominantly spinal or osteoarticular any bone may be involved, with single or multiple lesions. Definitive diagnosis from biopsy may be difficult as culture from bone specimens is often negative and histology, although indicative of chronic inflammatory tissue, may be non-specific.

Treatment should be started as soon as there is radiological and clinical suspicion and before deformity with crippling long-term disabilities arises. At the Red Cross Hospital in Cape Town about 50 children under the age of 12 years are seen each year. The sites predominently involved are:

1. Spine, 65%–70%. (This figure is similar to figures from India and Asia, but is 15%–20% higher than reported from Europe[1,2].)
2. Osteo articular (large joints), 20%–25%.
3. Tubular bones and flat bones, 10%–15%.

Spinal TB

The imaging features by plain X-ray[3-6], CT[7-12] and MR[13-16] have been well documented. The disease is most commonly reported in the thoracolumbar region[1]. The cervical spine is an exception to the indolent nature of lesions as pain occurs relatively early with torticollis a dominant and cosmetically obvious feature[17].

The common site of origin is within the vertebral body near the vertebral end plates. The involvement of the intervertebral disc is a secondary process. The disc has two components, a surrounding outer annulus fibrosis and an inner fluid nucleus pulposis. The annulus is relatively avascular in adults and this may provide some initial barrier to infection. In young children it is more vascularized[2,14,18] and relatively early disc space narrowing occurs when plain films show vertebral body involvement. The MR findings will be discussed later on page 86, but they show that the disc and particularly its nucleus pulposis component remain comparatively intact even in advanced disease. The disc or its remnants are displaced into the affected vertebral bodies, causing implosive destruction and further disintegration[15,16] (Fig. 6.1a,b,c).

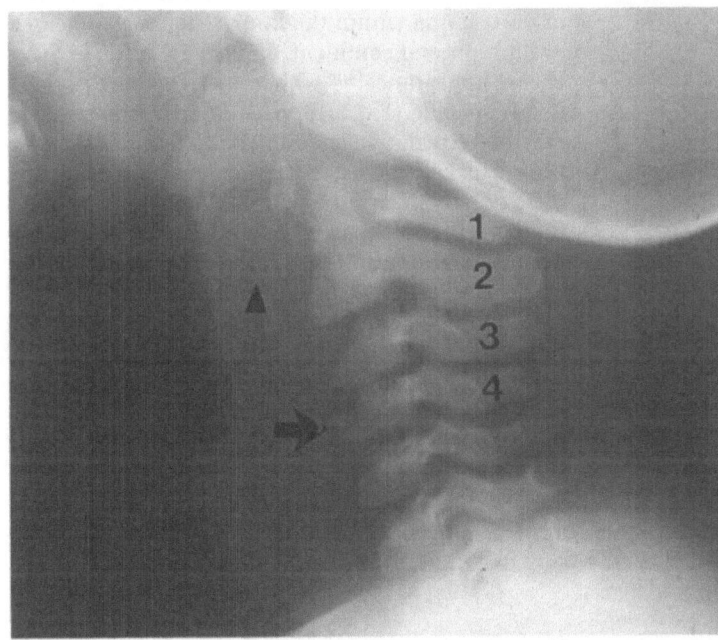

Fig. 6.1. a Lateral X-ray in a 2-year old child, with early involvement of body of C4 (arrow). The anterior bevelling of the body of C3 is normal at this age. Cervical gland calcification is present (arrow head). **b** CT showing early lytic changes in body of C4. Calcified nodes noted (arrow). **c** Sagittal T2 MR showing increased signal in body of C4. Anterior abscess is forming. Nucleus pulposis retains its normal high signal.

a

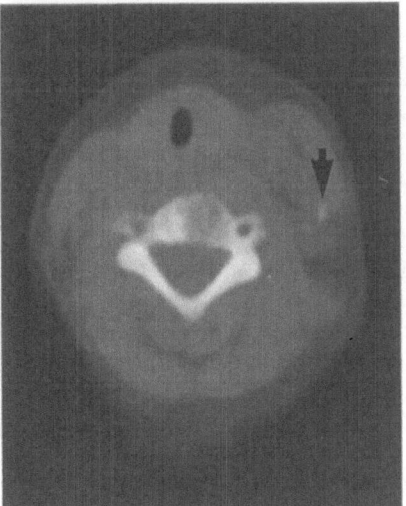

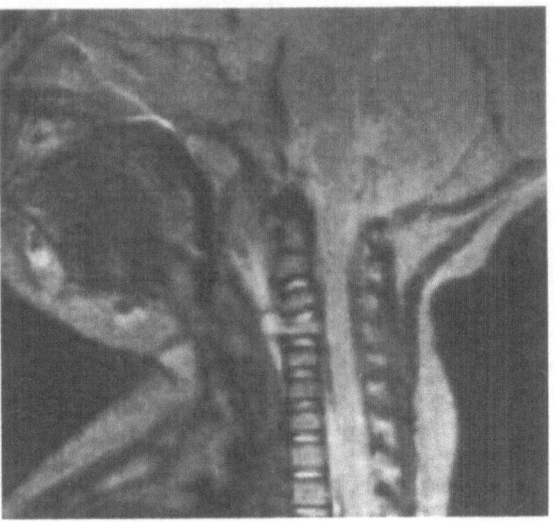

b   c

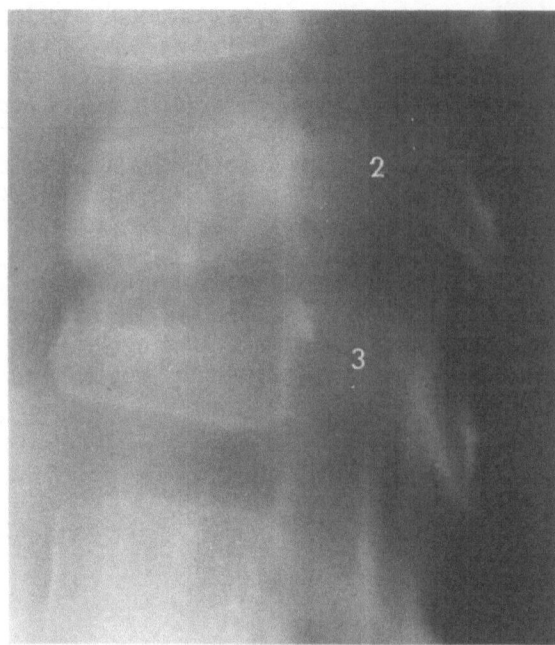

Fig. 6.2. Lateral tomogram of L2-L3 with early collapse of the body of L3, lytic destruction in the bodies of L2 and L3 and disc space narrowing.

There may also be little initial visible change in the vertebral body, but lateral tomography can be utilized to show the lytic destructive changes (Fig. 6.2). The lateral X-ray or tomogram may also be used to note the number of vertebrae involved by counting the posterior elements (Fig. 6.3a). The destructive process extends through the vertebra, resulting in collapse with characteristic anterior wedging. The extruded caseous material causes both anterior and posterior tuberculous abscesses with spread of the disease under the spinal ligaments (Fig. 6.3b,c). The tuberculous abscess may cause an aneurysmal defect[19] (similar to the erosion caused by aortic aneurysm) on the anterior surface of the vertebra (Fig. 6.4a,b,c). In the frontal projection, involvement of pedicles can be noted and paraspinal soft tissue swelling can be seen (Fig. 6.5a,b). Large paraspinal abscesses are a feature of spinal TB and their presence can also be detected by ultrasound (Fig. 6.6a,b).

The diagnosis of spinal TB is not always easy[5] and the appearances may vary in different countries and races[5,6]. The imaging appearances must be fitted into appropriate clinical settings. In adults, preservation of the disc space has been reported[20,21], but this must be uncommon in the presence of vertebral collapse[5]. In pyogenic infection pain is an early

feature and proteolytic enzymes affect the disc to cause early narrowing. Histiocytosis causes early vertebral collapse but the disc space is usually well preserved and the diagnosis may be assisted by the finding of well circumscribed lesions elsewhere in the skeleton. Neoplasms, usually secondary, may cause more sclerosis and the disc space is preserved. The characteristic features of CT and particularly MR are both very helpful in establishing the diagnosis.

Computed Tomography

The early changes of spinal TB consist of lytic areas of destruction within the body. They may be single or multiple and confluent, and have a cystic or Swiss cheese appearance[12,16] which, though characteristic, is not specific (Fig 6.4b, 6.7). Similar appearances may be seen in pyogenic infection, lymphoma, histiocytosis and metastasis. Fragmentation and complete destruction of the vertebral body occurs when the body implodes (Fig. 6.8a). The result is high-density debris within paravertebral collections (Fig. 6.8b). The posterior extension can be seen in axial sections, and symptoms of spinal cord compression result when there is intra-spinal canal narrowing of approximately 50%–60%[15]. Pedicle destruction and posterior element involvement that is not apparent on plain radiography is well demonstrated by CT (Figs 6.4b, 6.8a,b). CT will also show the size of abscesses (Fig. 6.9a) and CT-guided needle aspiration may be used to drain an abscess, causing compression in confined spaces (Fig. 6.9b).

Magnetic Resonance Imaging

The early bone lesions in spinal TB give a vertebral body T1-hypointense and a T2-hyperintense signal[15,16]. The changes are well seen on sagittal T2 images. These MR images reflect the pathological features recorded by Campere and Garrison[22]. The nucleus pulposis, being of a fluid nature, gives a bright T2 signal which is initially preserved (Fig. 6.10). As the disease progresses the disc or its remnants are plunged or driven into the weakened vertebral body (Figs 6.11, 6.12, 6.13d).

The destruction of the vertebral body by this internal implosion causes complete collapse with the spread of pus, bony fragments, and disc material in all directions[16]. MR, with its multiplanar capacity, demonstrates well the extent of the disease and the extradural intraspinal cord compression that causes

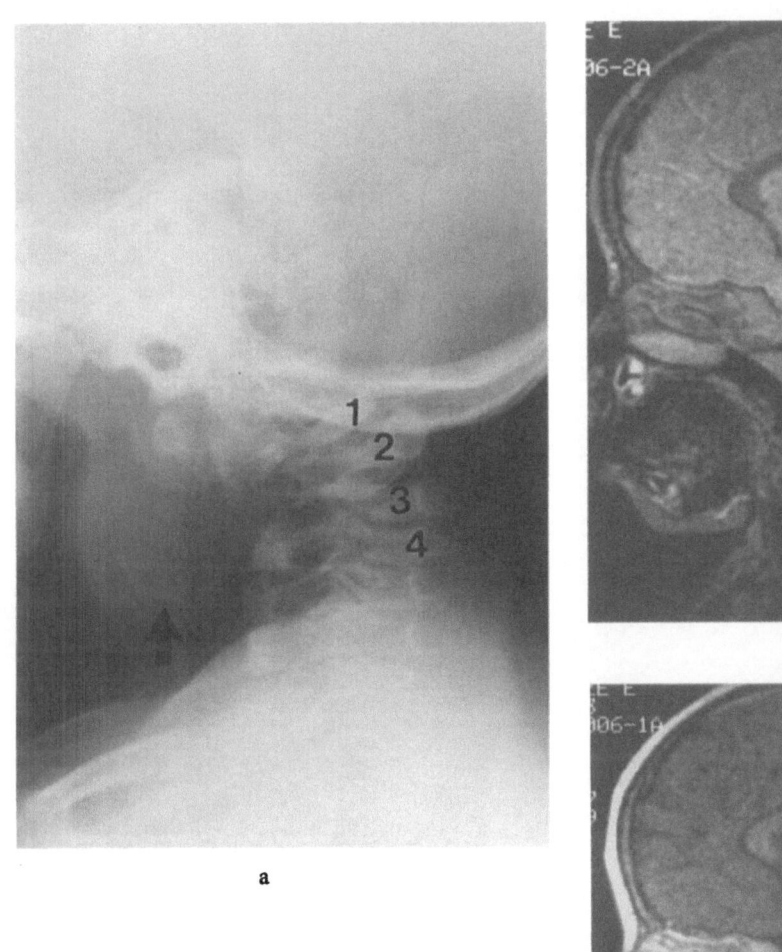

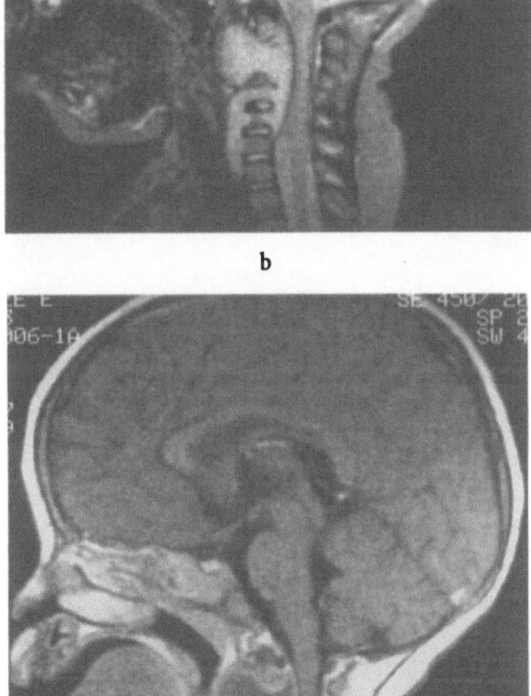

Fig. 6.3. a Destruction of the bodies of C2-C4 with calcific debris in anterior abscess (arrow). b Sagittal T2 MR demonstrating destruction of C2-C4 with anterior and posterior abscesses. c Same case sagittal T1 MR with IV gadolinium enhancement. Peripheral enhancement with non-enhancing necrotic content of abscess.

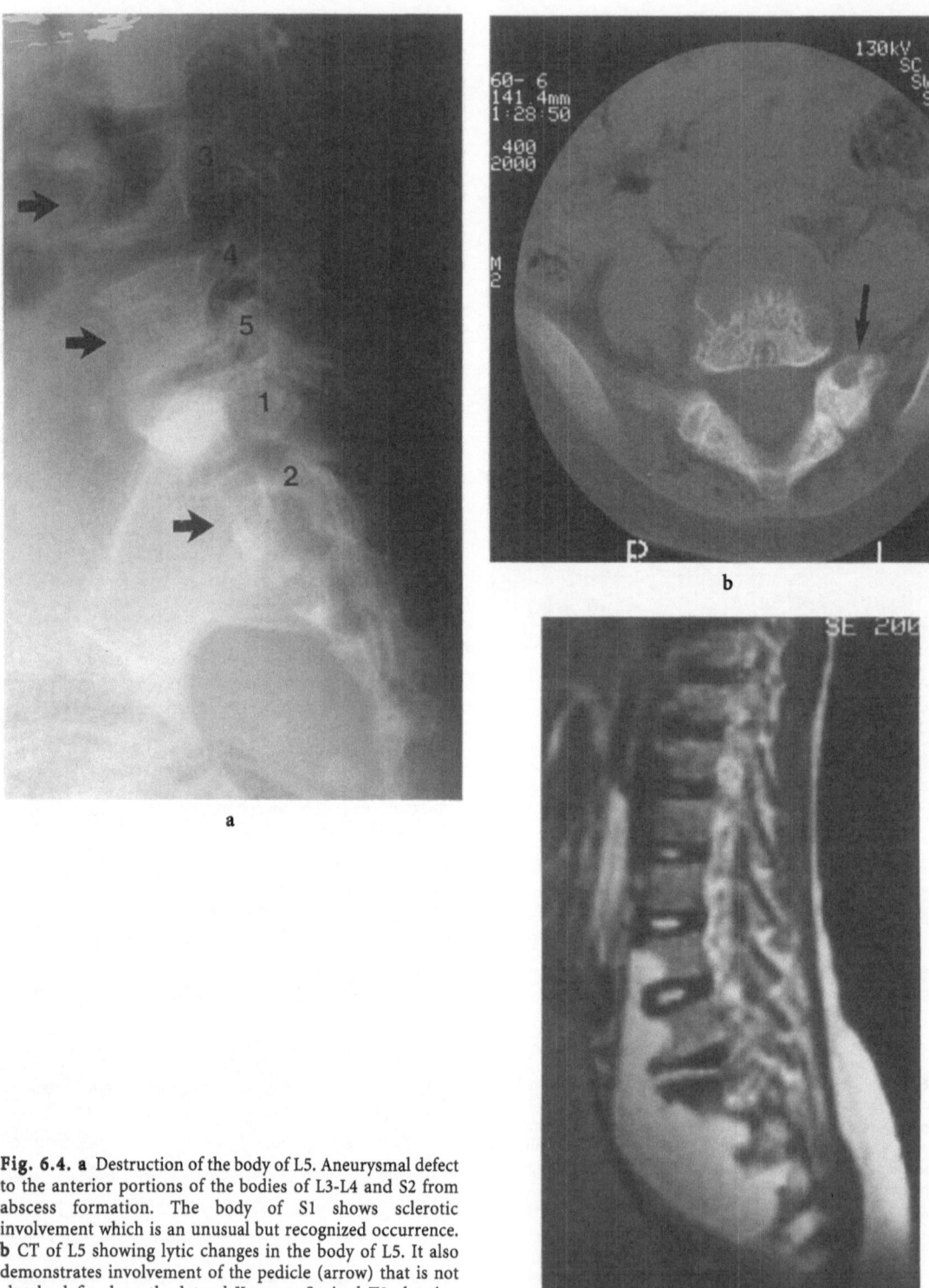

Fig. 6.4. a Destruction of the body of L5. Aneurysmal defect
to the anterior portions of the bodies of L3-L4 and S2 from
abscess formation. The body of S1 shows sclerotic
involvement which is an unusual but recognized occurrence.
b CT of L5 showing lytic changes in the body of L5. It also
demonstrates involvement of the pedicle (arrow) that is not
clearly defined on the lateral X-ray. **c** Sagittal T2 showing
large anterior abscess, causing aneurysmal defect in C3-C4
and S2.

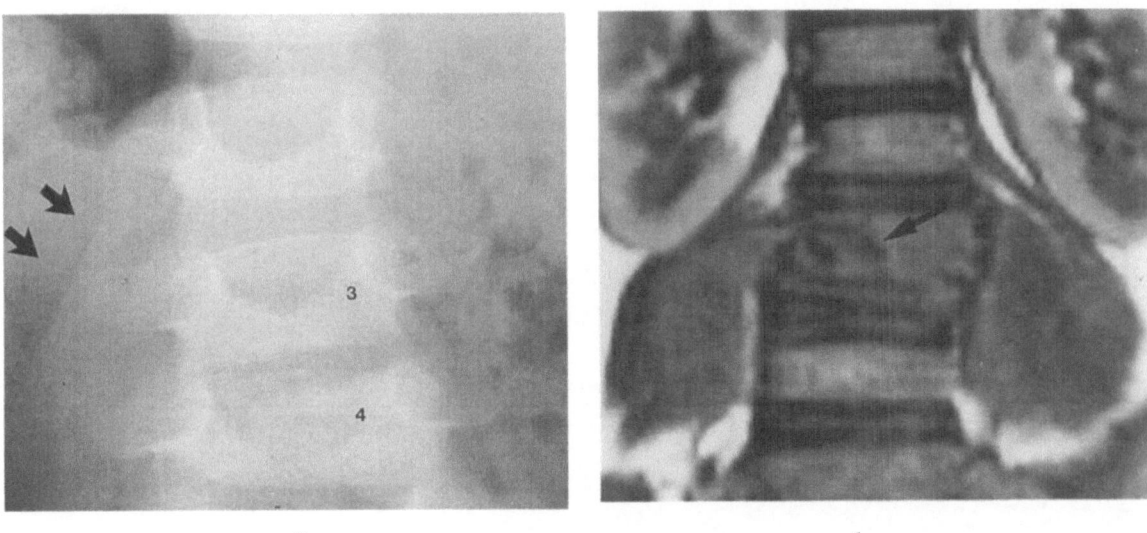

a   b

Fig. 6.5. a Frontal X-ray showing early collapse of the R side of the body of L4 and involvement of the pedicle. The psoas abscess is demonstrated (arrow). **b** Comparable coronal T1 MR showing vertebral body destruction (arrow) and large bilateral psoas abscesses.

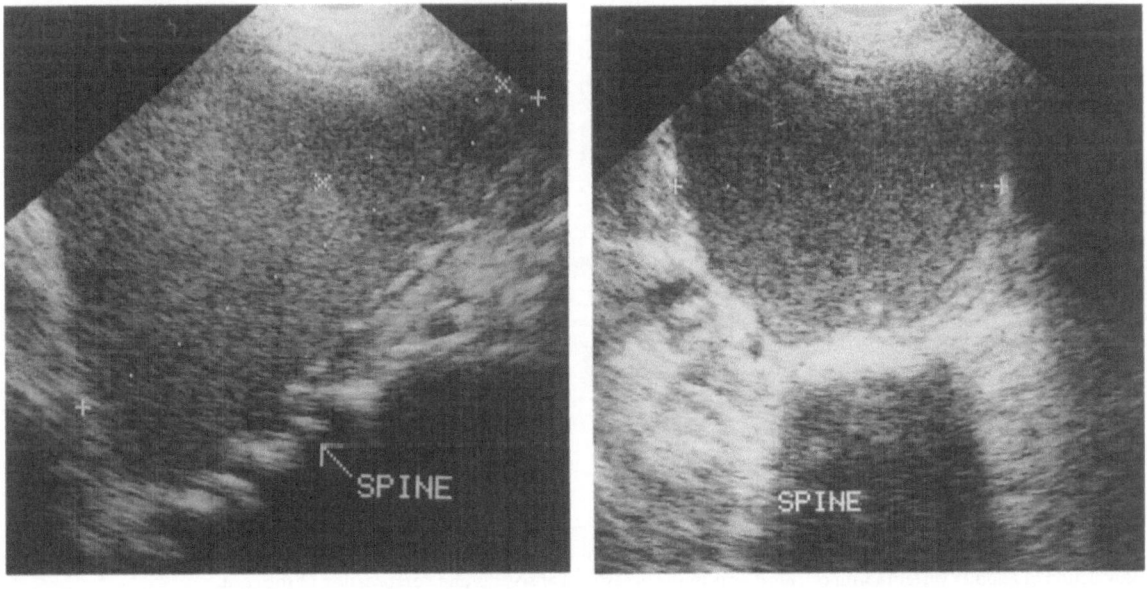

a   b

Fig. 6.6. a Lateral US showing irregular vertebral body (arrow) and a large anterior spinal abscess. **b** Transverse US of the same case.

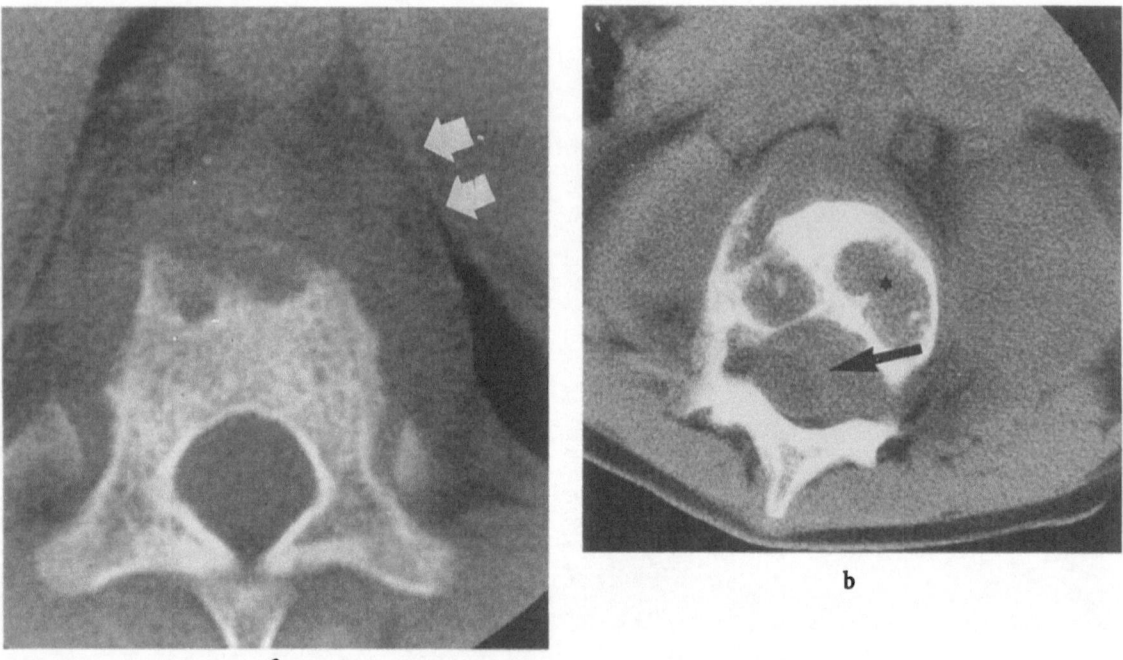

Fig. 6.7. a CT showing lytic "cystic" destruction of anterior body and anterior spinal abscess (arrows). **b** More extensive cystic destruction (asterisk) as disc material intrudes into the body. A posterior abscess is encroaching on the spinal canal (arrow).

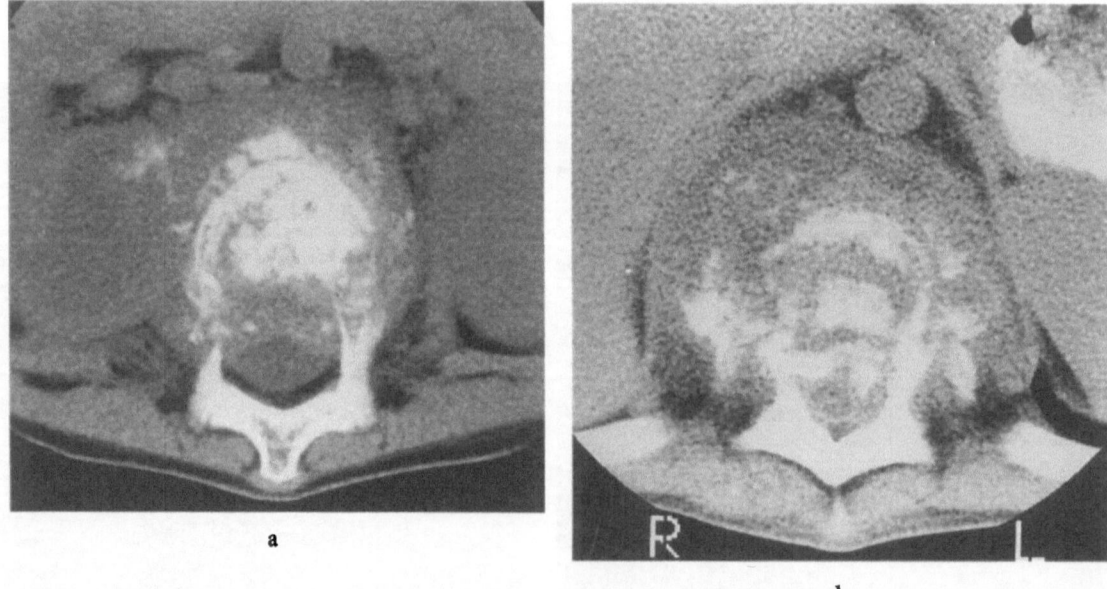

Fig. 6.8. a Implosion of the vertebral body with involvement of the posterior elements on both sides. **b**(same case) More complete destruction of another vertebra with calcific debris in the paraspinal abscesses and compression of the cord.

Potts paraplegia (Figs 6.10–6.13). MR also demonstrates the involvement of posterior elements adjoining spinous (Fig. 6.12a) and transverse processes and ribs, which are not well seen by plain radiography, and may also demonstrate involvement of unsuspected vertebrae (Figs 6.13b,c,d).

In TB, the disc nucleus retains its normal T2 signal until late, whilst in pyogenic infection there is an early decreased T1 signal and an increased T2 signal from the body and disc space[14,18,23]. Variation in hydration of the nucleus has also been noted in nonspecific discitis with an early decrease in T1 and an

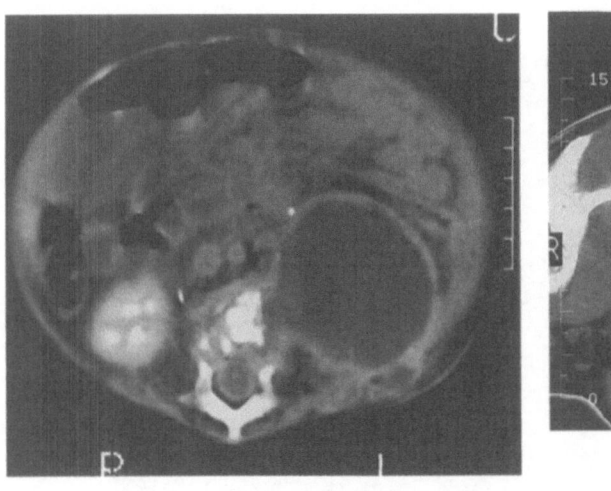

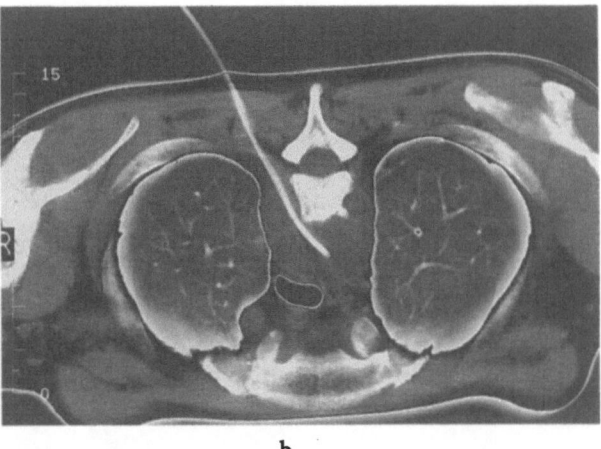

b

a

Fig. 6.9. a CT showing large left psoas abscess which has displaced the R kidney. There is also abscess anterior to the affected vertebral body. **b** CT guided drainage of an anterior thoracic abscess which was causing tracheal compression. Destruction of the vertebral body is seen.

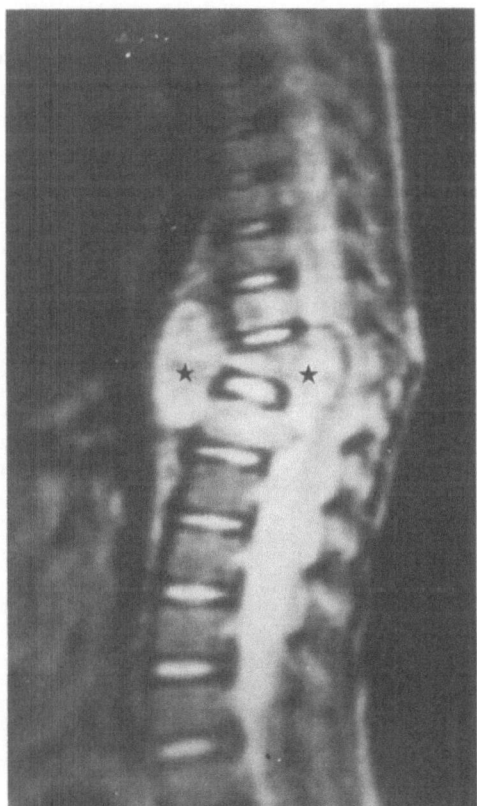

Fig. 6.10. Sagittal T2 MR. The bodies of T1–T3 are involved, with a high intensity signal. The nucleus pulposis of the vertebral discs retain their high signal and the body of T2 is collapsing with its adjacent lower disc plunging into it. Anterior and posterior abscesses are present (asterisks).

increase in T2, followed by reversal of this appearance at a later stage[24].

Pott's Paraplegia

This is the most serious complication of TB spondylitis. It is due to compression of the spinal cord by the extradural mass of tuberculous debris. It occurs when the intra-spinal space is compromised by over 50%–60%[15]. It is also influenced by the severe angulation and kyphosis which stretches the cord over the angulation and intra-spinal mass. CT has been used in its evaluation[8,11], and we have compared the usefulness of plain radiography, CT and MR in its management[15,16]. CT gives good appreciation of the amount of bone destruction[9,11,15,16]. This is important if stabilizing surgery at a later stage is contemplated. The relative effectiveness of conservative treatment as advocated by Konstam[25] of Nigeria or of surgical intervention as practised by Hodgson[26] of Hong Kong is debatable and is the subject of ongoing MRC trials[27]. Orthopedic surgeons in Cape Town follow the conservative approach[28] and Potts paraplegia is assessed by both CT and MR. Although CT gives a good appreciation of the bony destruction and spinal canal narrowing, it is limited by its axial capacity. All cases with neurological signs have an MR with sagittal and axial scans for preliminary assessment. Anti-tuberculous drug therapy is em-

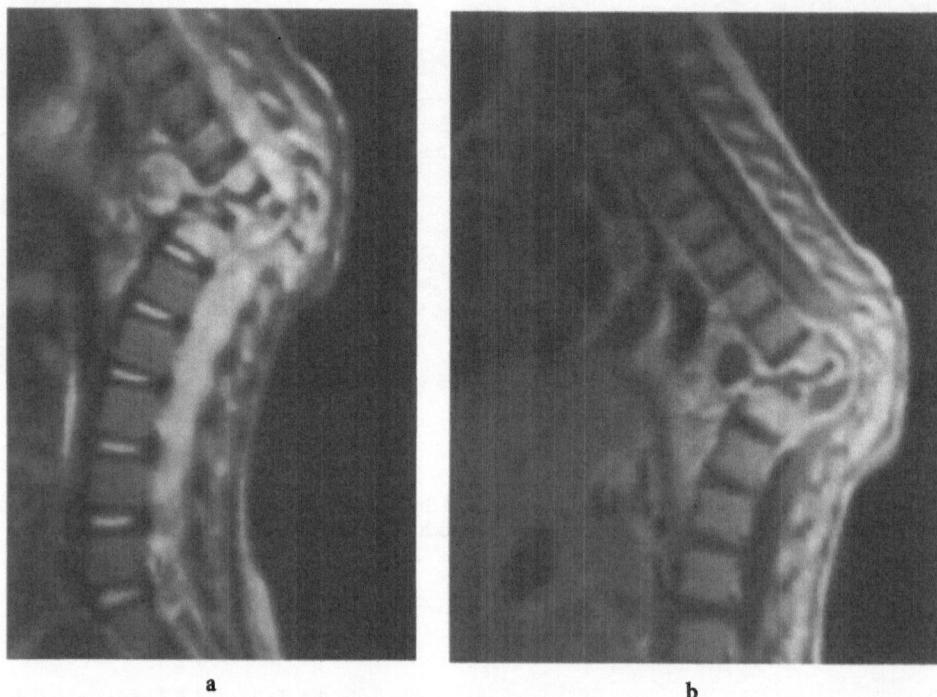

a   b

Fig. 6.11. a Sagittal T2 MR. The bodies of T9 and T12 show high intensity signals. The bodies of T10–T11 have been destroyed, the intervening disc nuclei have retained their signals and are plunged into the bodies. Large anterior and posterior abscesses have formed. **b** Same case T1 MR IV gadolinium-enhanced showing enhancing inflammatory tissue with non-enhancing necrotic content.

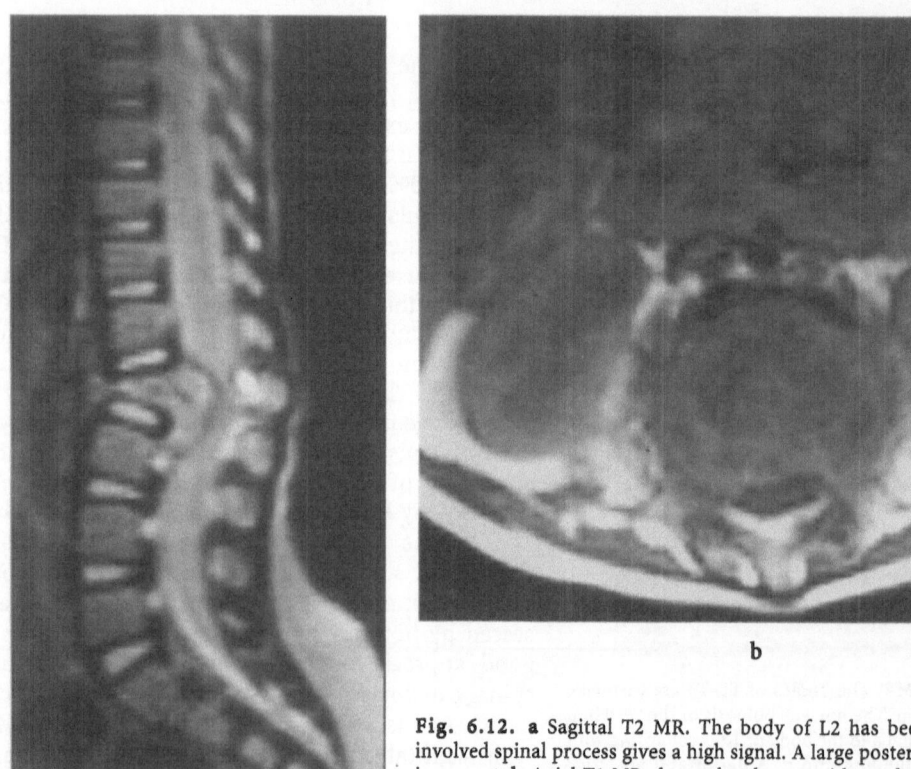

b

Fig. 6.12. a Sagittal T2 MR. The body of L2 has been destroyed and the involved spinal process gives a high signal. A large posterior extradural abscess is present. **b** Axial T1 MR shows the abscess with marked compression of the spinal cord.

a

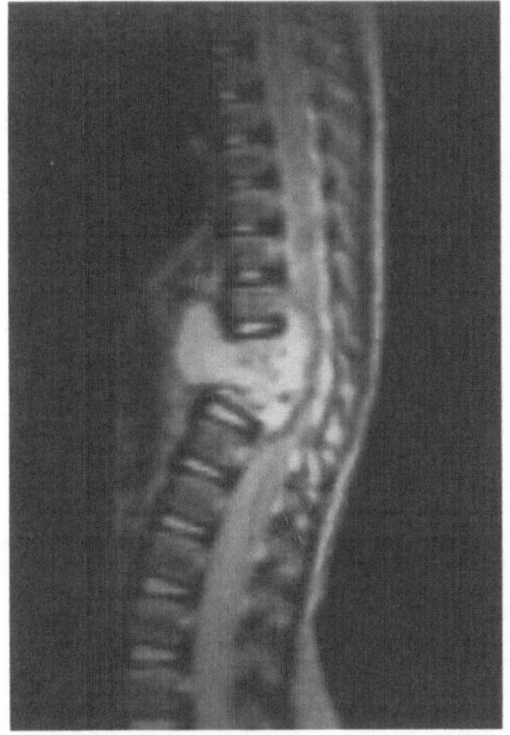
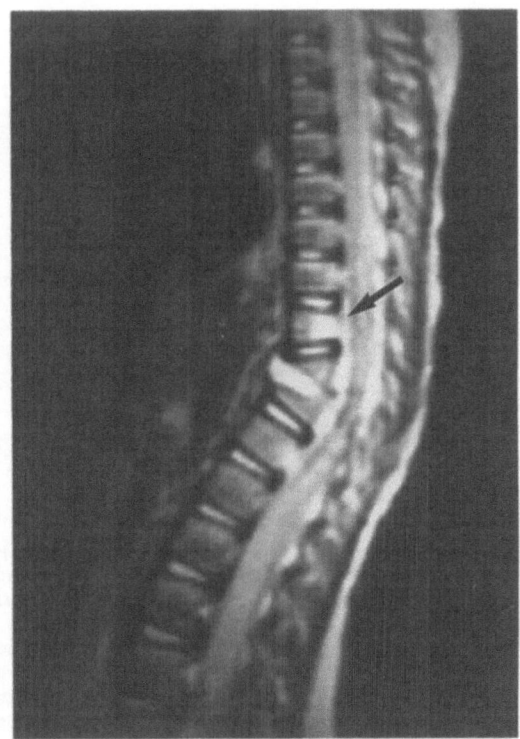

a

b

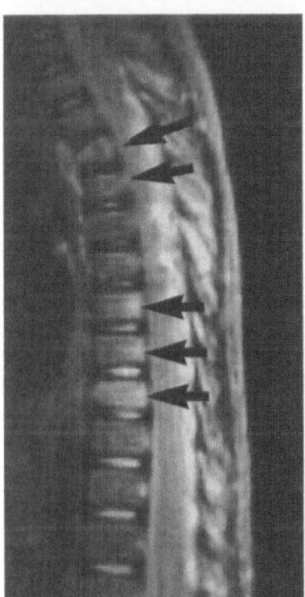
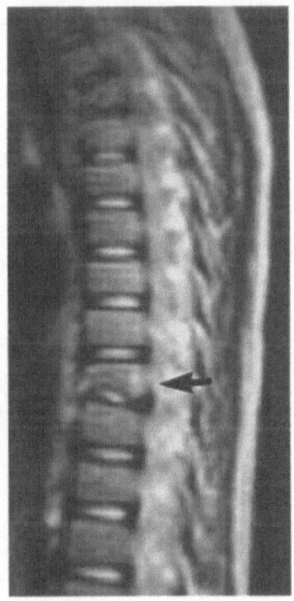

c

d

Fig. 6.13. a Sagittal T2 MR showing complete destruction of the bodies of T10–T11. Anterior and posterior high signal abscesses are present. b Sagittal T2 MR. After 3 months anti-TB drug therapy the abscesses have resolved but unsuspected involvement of the body of T9 is now demonstrated (arrow). The child made a complete neurological recovery. c This case (same as shown in Fig. 6.30) had skull TB and a barely discernible T3 body lesion on plain X-ray. Sagittal T2 MR showed involvement of T3 (arrow) with an anterior abscess but also unsuspected involvement of T4 and the bodies of T8,9,10 (arrow heads). d Sagittal T2 MR. After 3 months anti-TB treatment the lesions are healing and disc nucleus intrusion is seen in the lower body of T9 (arrow).

barked on for 3 months and if there is no improvement, another MR is performed prior to contemplated surgical decompression. MR features the extradural mass as either predominantly "pus" with high T2 signal or predominantly "granulation" tissue with an intermediate T2 signal[15]. The "pus" cases are expected to respond to conservative management and not to need decompressive surgery (Fig. 6.13a,b).

Finally, modern imaging should aim to provide the clinician with the following information.

1. The number of vertebrae involved, for which plain radiography may be adequate but has limitations. Extensive disease is best studied by CT and MR.

2. The severity of bone destruction, about which plain X-rays give a workable visualization, but

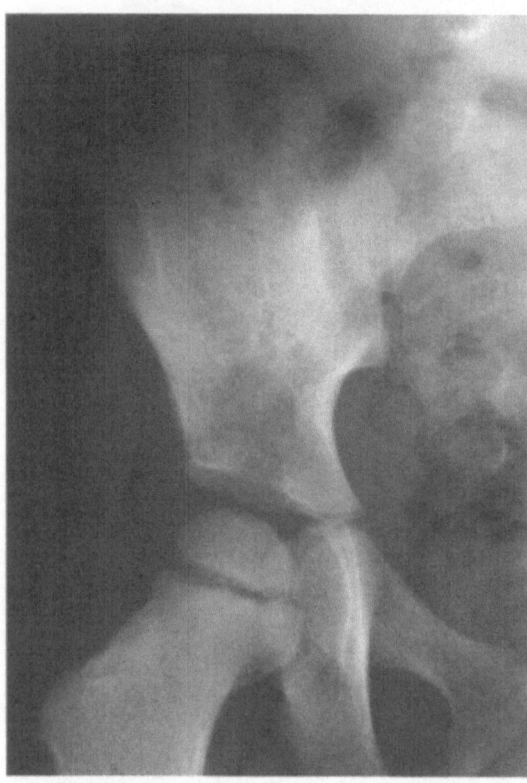

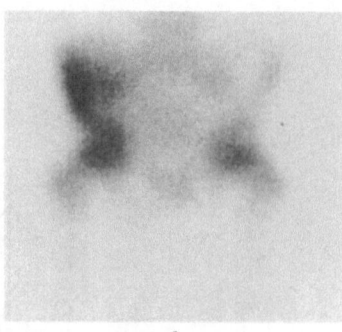

a

b

Fig. 6.14. a "Normal hip", i.e., cystic changes in acetabulum but normal joint space. **b** Isotope scan shows iliac involvement is more extensive than seen on X-ray. **c** Cystic changes in acetabulum and "protrusio acetabulum" type of deformity. **d** Early "Perthes"- like changes causing collapse of femoral head. **e,f** (same case) **e** CT shows destructive changes in femoral head and hip joint. **f** Coronal T1 MR showing loss of signal in lateral side of head and also showing more extensive changes in iliac bone. **g** Cystic changes in hip bones with gross destruction of the femoral head.

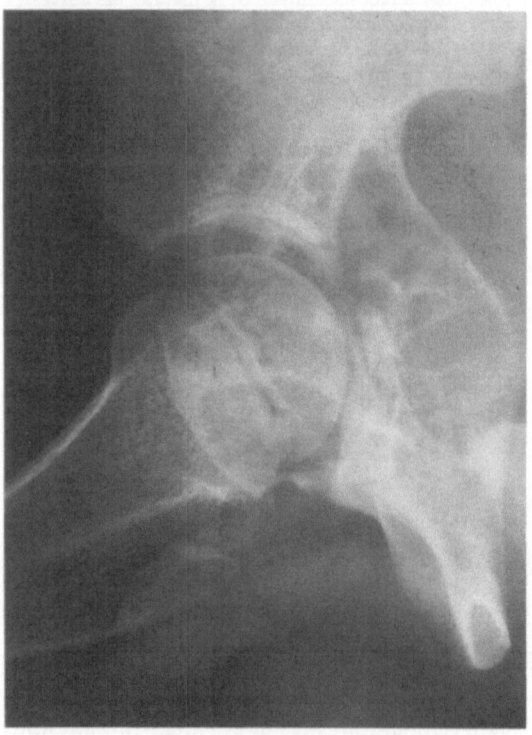

c

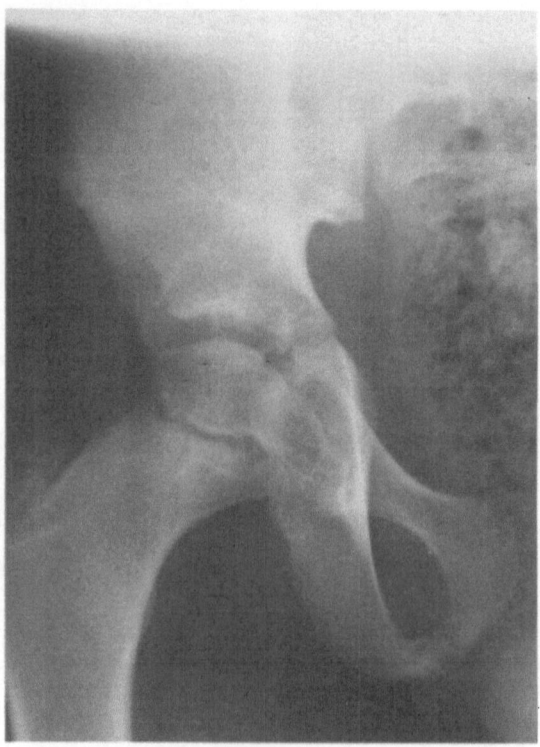

d

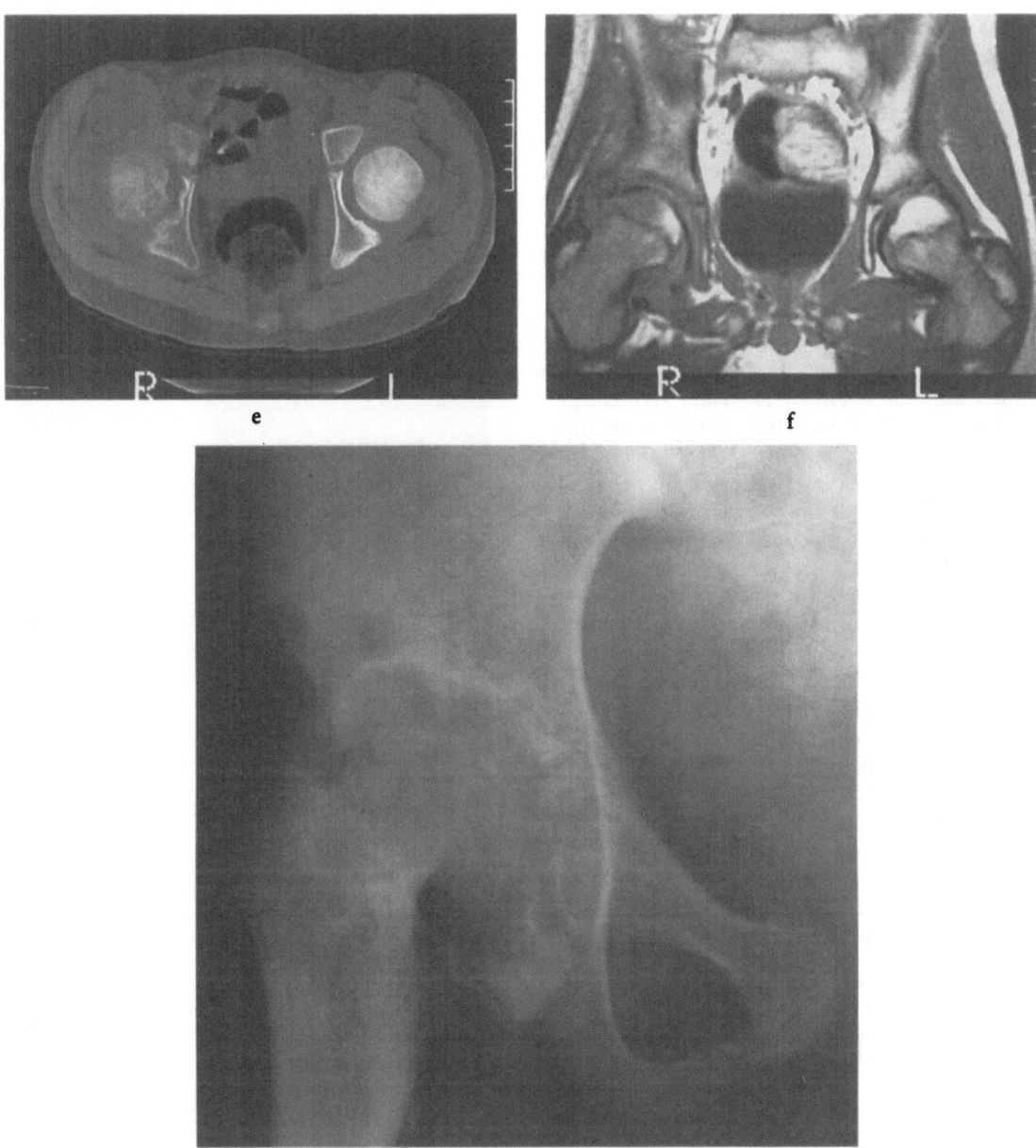

e   f

g

Fig. 6.14. (*continued*)

CT or MR may show the disease to be more extensive. Early infection may only be seen by MR.

3. The site of involvement within the vertebra, best seen by MR and CT. The degree of bone destruction, especially posterior element involvement, which is common in established disease, is best appreciated by CT, although subtle marrow changes may be first seen on MR.

4. The angle of kyphosis which can be well measured on lateral plain X-ray although lateral tomography may be necessary.

5. Soft tissue involvement of paraspinal abscesses and disc sequestration, which is best evaluated by MR.

6. The extent of cord compression may be estimated both by CT nd MR, but MR is the best modality, and if available, should be used in preference to myelography in all cases of cord involvement.

Osteo-articular Lesions

Joint involvement is considered to be initially an ef-
fusive condition[1]. Infection may result from synovial lesions directly affecting the joint, or from a
metaphyseal infection spreading into the joint
cavity. Without treatment, there will be destruction
of articular surfaces, obliteration of joint spaces,
abscess formation and sinuses with the end result of
fibrous or bony ankylosis. The disease is most frequent in the large joints, particularly the weight-
bearing hips and knees, but also occurs in the
shoulder and elbow joints. The early radiographic
signs may be difficult to detect. The synovial infection features a hyperemic osteopenia of the bones
and the joint space may be initially blurred and
eventually narrowed, as the increased pressure com-
pounds cartilage destruction. The progression is
from caseous osteitis to fragmentation and destruction of the joint and the prognosis ultimately
depends on the amount of joint preservation. In the
hip, progressive destruction of subarticular bones
will cause cystic lesions on both sides of the joint.
A clinico-radiological classification based on
gross architectural changes has been compiled by
Shanmugasundaram[1]. Five types were noted in children with the implication that conservative treatment was more likely to be successful in the first
three.

1. "Normal" (minimal joint space narrowing, but
   cystic changes in bones) (Fig. 6.14a,b).

2. "Protruso-acetabuli" (cystic medial ballooning
   of the acetabuli) (Fig. 6.14c).

3. "Perthes" type (fragmentation of femoral head)
   (Fig. 6.14d,e,f).

4. "Travelling acetabuli" (progressive upward displacement of femoral head).

5. "Dislocating hip" (posterior dislocation).

This type of descriptive analysis is mainly of help
to orthopedic surgeons in assessing prognosis but
any gross destruction of either femoral head
or joint (Fig. 6.14g) must obviously impair the
prognosis.

In the knee joint, the disease is predominantly
synovial[30] and in the early stages differentiation
from monoarticular rheumatoid arthritis may be
difficult (Fig. 6.15). Marginal erosions of the bone at
the attachment of synovial membrane are a feature

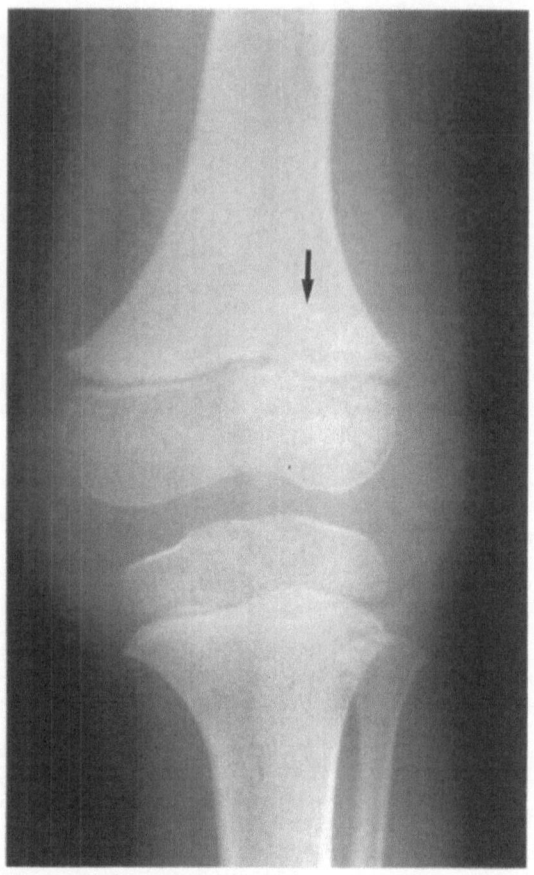

Fig. 6.15. Swollen knee joint with accentuated growth of
femoral and tibial epiphyses. Monarticular rheumatoid arthritis
and hemophilia (before joint destruction) can give similar appearances; clue to diagnosis is faint sclerosis and cystic change in
the femoral metaphysis (arrow).

in adults that we have not noted in children.
Eventually cystic lesions tend to develop and may
extend through the epiphyses into the metaphyses
(Fig. 6.16). In the foot, cystic changes may be seen in
the tarsal bones (Fig. 6.17).

In the upper limb the shoulder joint is commonly
affected. Two types of changes at the glenohumeral
joint may be seen. In the exudative form, progressive features of synovitis predominate, with associated demineralization, soft tissue swelling,
marginal erosions and eventual joint and bone destruction with cavity formation (Fig. 6.18a). In the
dry type, "caries sicca", atrophic changes occur
(Fig. 6.18b). At the elbow joint any of the three
bones may be affected with some predilection for
the olecranon.

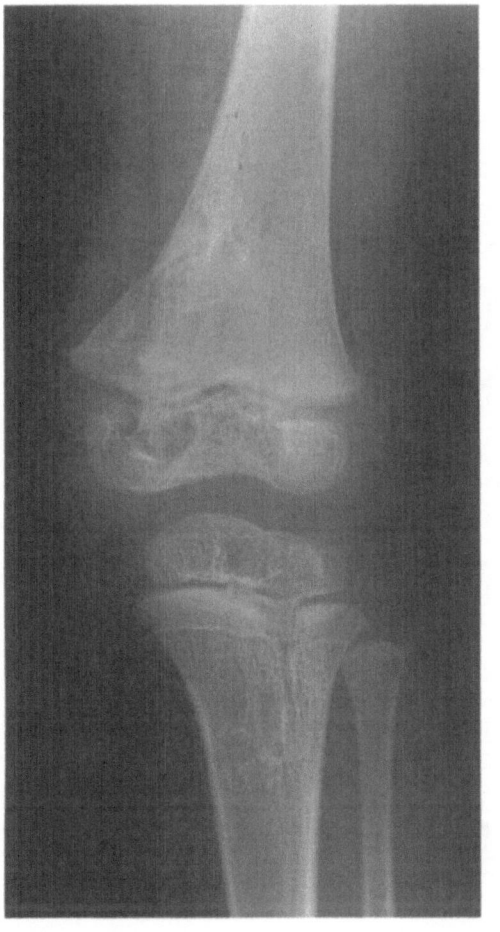 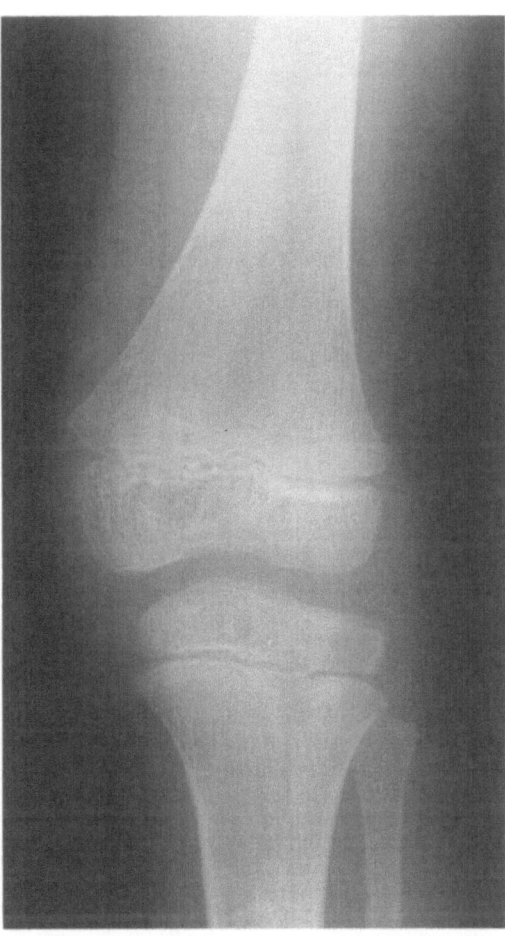

a   b

Fig. 6.16. a Cystic changes in femur and tibia with involvement of corresponding epiphyses. **b** 18 months after 6 months anti-TB treatment with progressive healing of lesions.

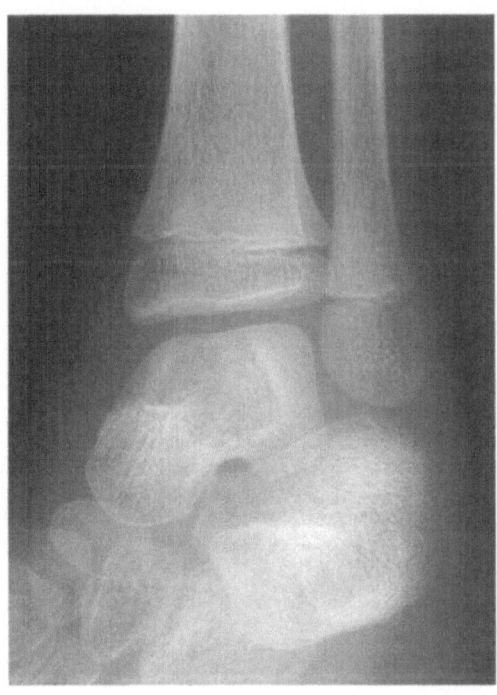

Fig. 6.17. Cystic lesion in talus.

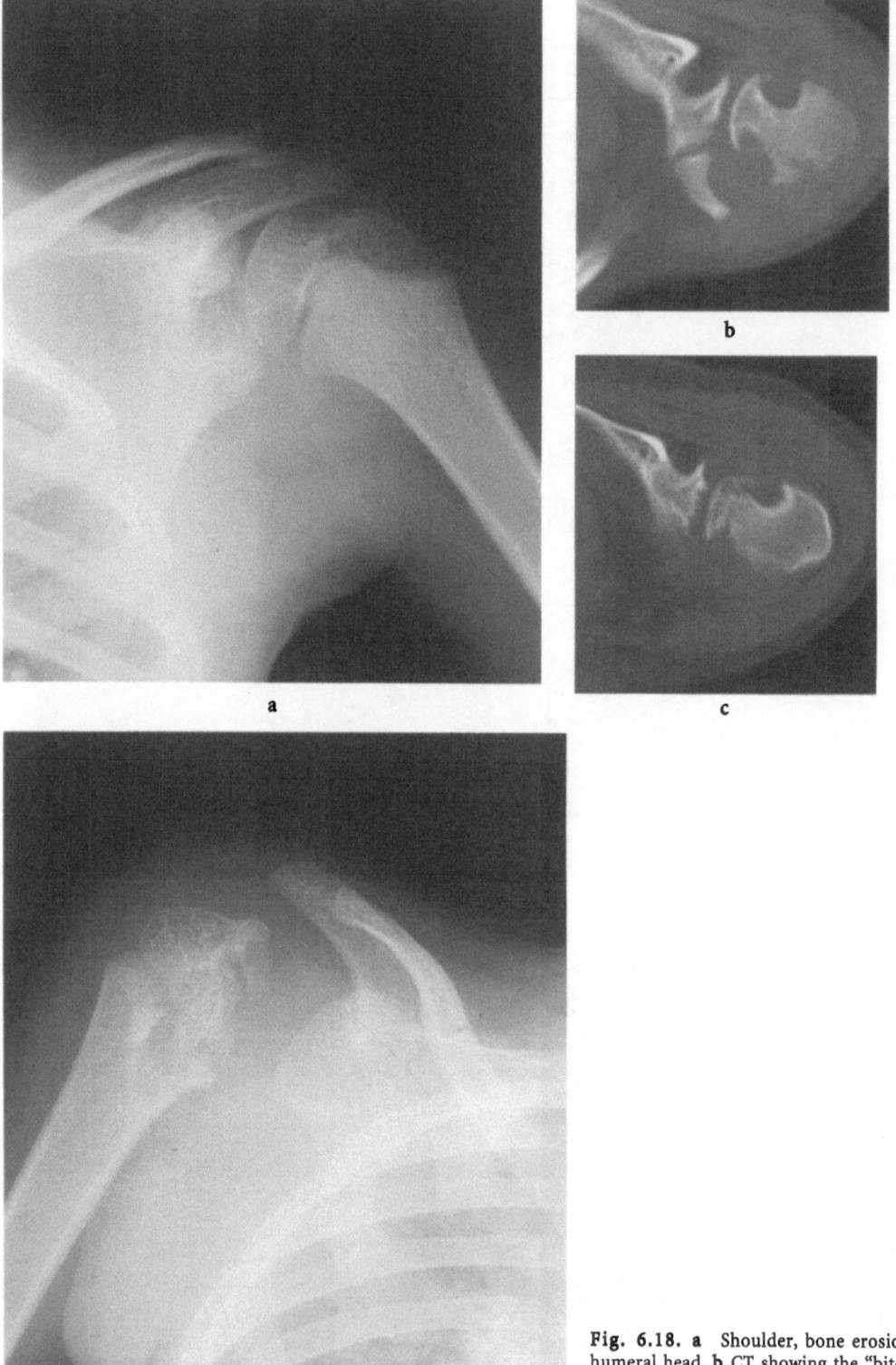

Fig. 6.18. a Shoulder, bone erosion in glenoid and humeral head. **b** CT showing the "bite" out of humeral head. **c** CT, a lower cut showing involved glenoid. **d** Extensive destruction of humeral head. This type of lesion is a precursor to "caries sicca".

Extra-articular Lesions

Tuberculous osteomyelitis occurred in other sites in about 10%–15% of our cases. It may involve any bone, but usually affects the long and short tubular bones, the flat bones of scapula, ribs and calvarium. In the tubular bones, the epiphysis (Fig. 6.19), metaphysis (Fig. 6.20) or both may be involved and the diaphysis (Fig. 6.21) may also be affected. The metaphysis is the commonest site and the features are of an indolent lytic destruction, often ill-defined, but sometimes circumscribed and usually with surrounding osteopenia, demineralization and soft tissue swelling. Periosteal reaction (Figs 6.20, 6.22) and sequestra are not common features, but may occur (Fig. 6.20). Sclerosis may be seen in long-standing cases (Fig. 6.23).

The common feature in the growing bones of children is that the proliferative destruction causes a cystic or expanded lesion. This is well seen in the flat bones of the scapula (Fig. 6.24), and in an extreme form as spina ventosa (from the Latin spina; a thorn-like process or projection: ventosa; inflated) in the phalanges (Fig. 6.25). Our use of MR was before suitable coils were available and the illustrations are not reproducible.

Multicystic forms occur in shafts of long bones (Fig. 6.26). They may involve multiple bones[31] and also involve the skull[32,33]. In the skull, TB often affects the fronto-parietal calvarium producing a round, lytic area, usually with an ill-defined border

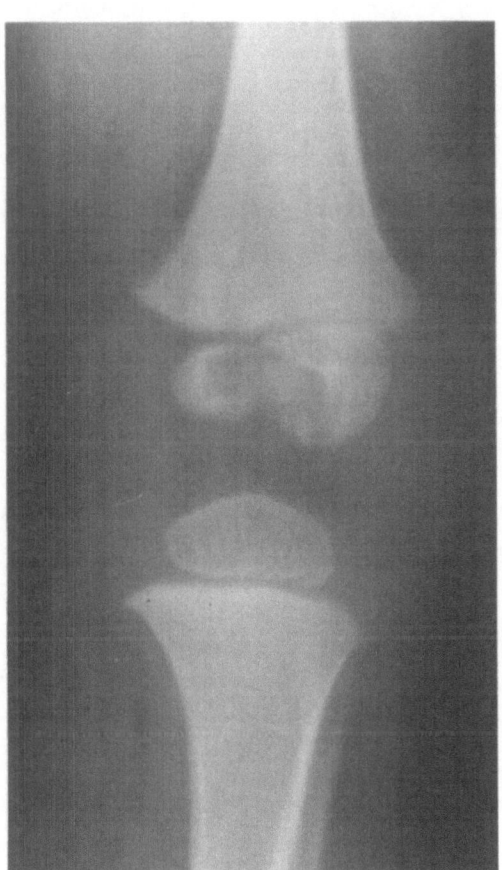

Fig. 6.19. Cystic lesion in femoral epiphysis.

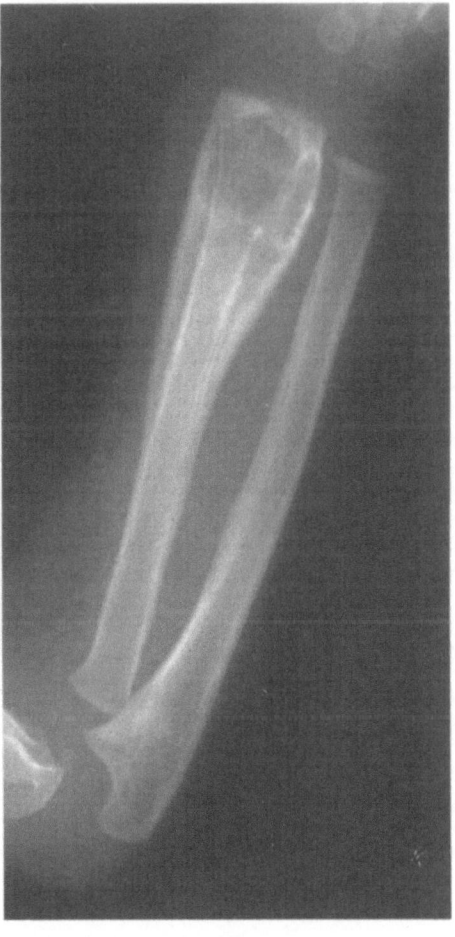

Fig. 6.20. Metaphyseal expanding lesion in distal radius. Sequestra formation is present.

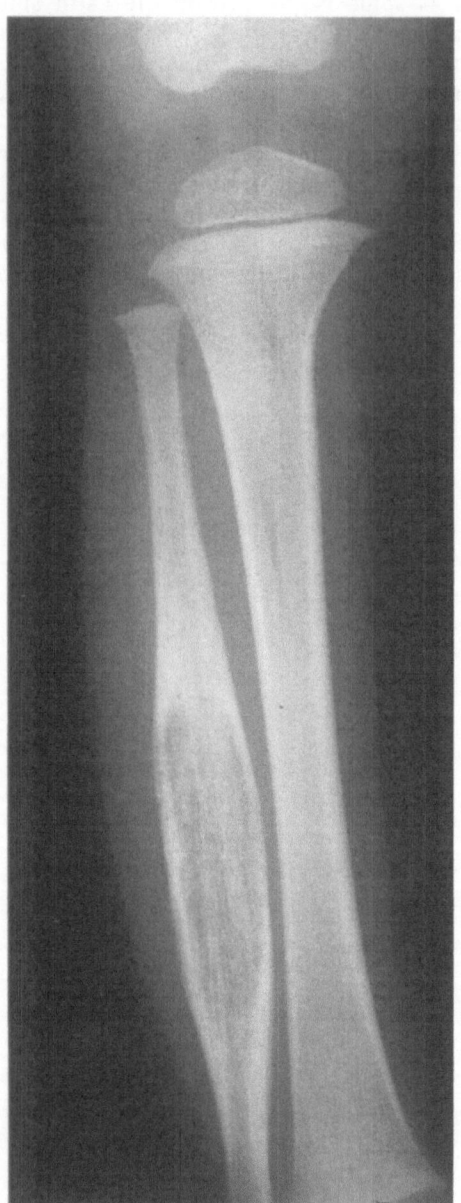

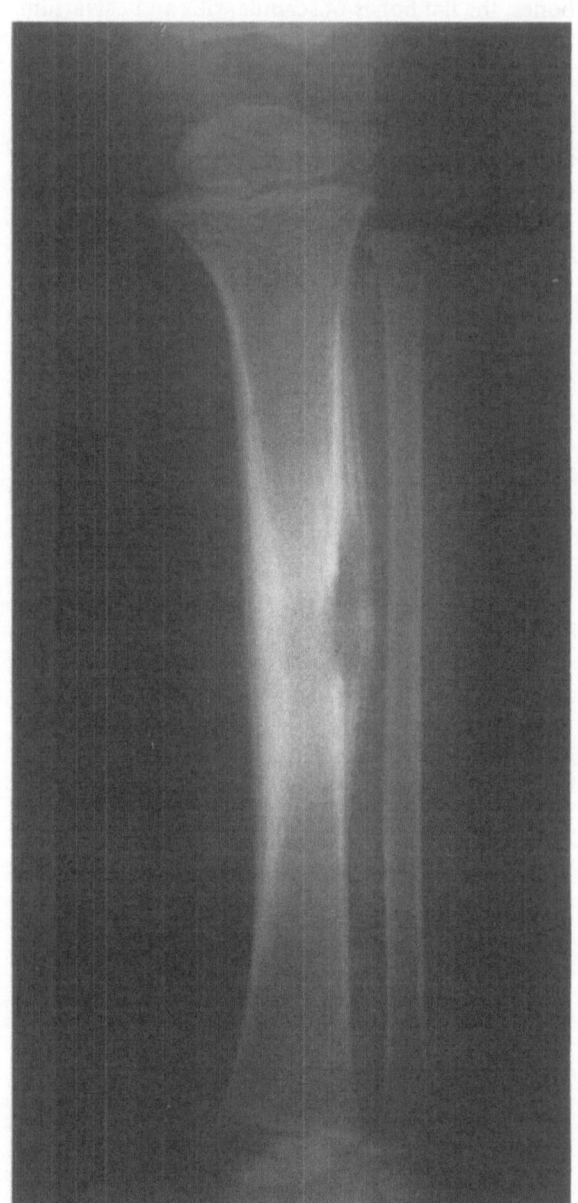

Fig. 6.21. Expansile lesion in diaphysis of fibula.

Fig. 6.22. Lesion in diaphysis of tibia giving periosteal reaction.

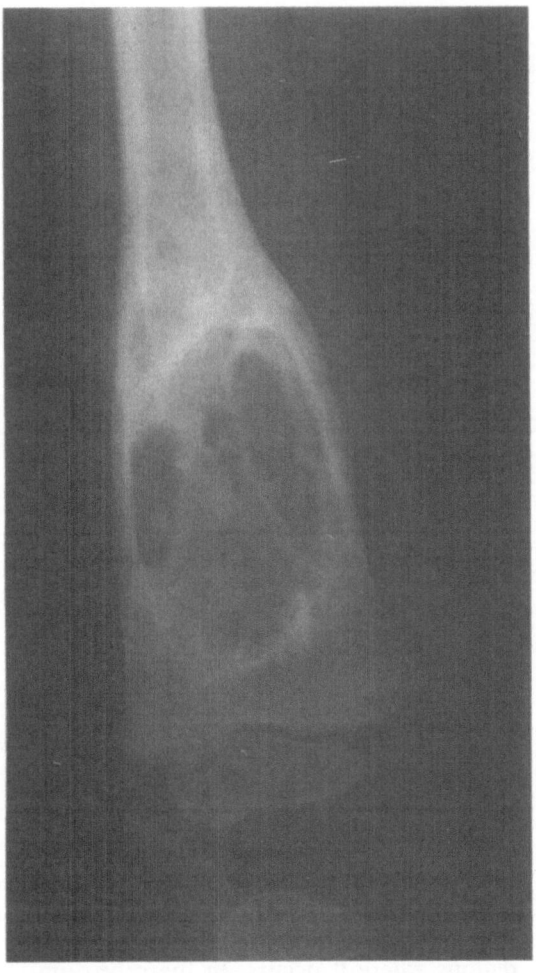

Fig. 6.23. Long-standing lesion in lower femur with considerable sclerosis.

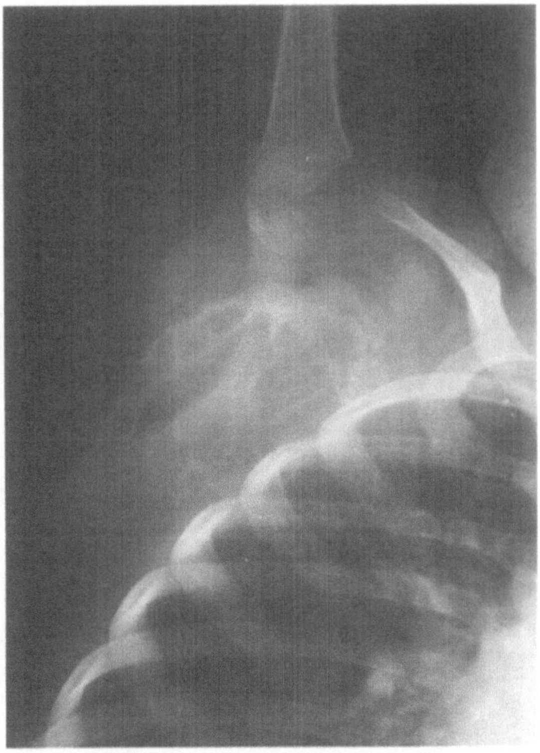

Fig. 6.24. Cytstic expansion of the scapula.

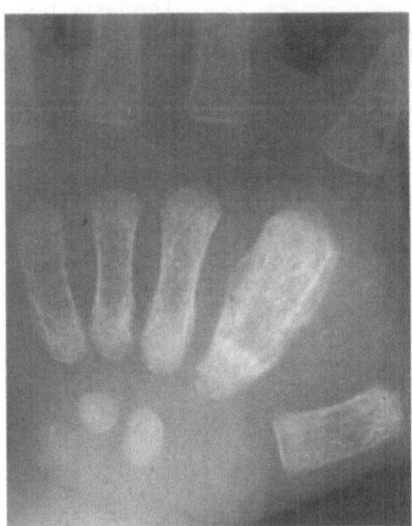

Fig. 6.25. "Spina ventosa" of a hand digit that was a completely painless lesion.

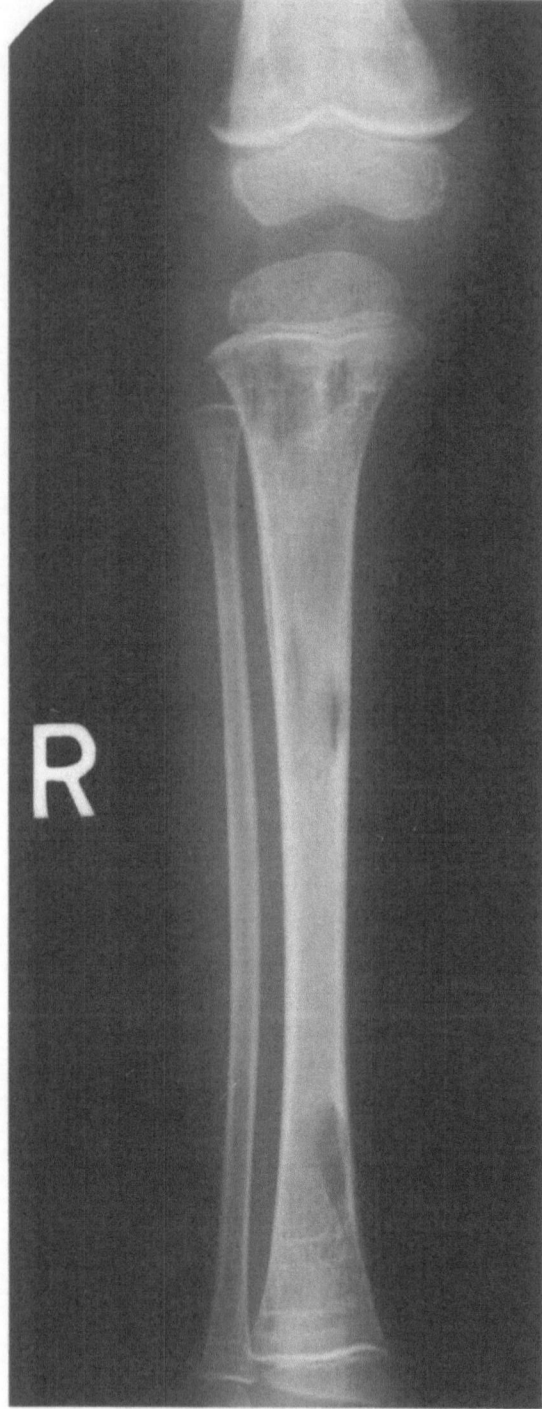

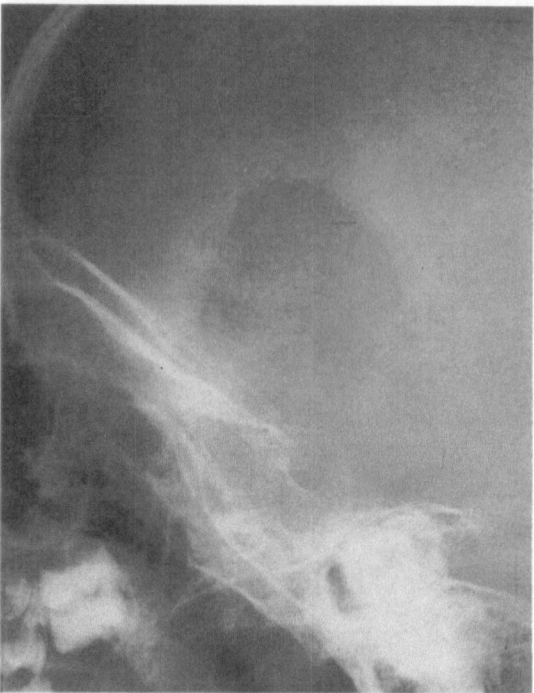

Fig. 6.27. Ill-defined lytic lesion in fronto-parietal area of skull.

(Fig. 6.27) which distinguishes it from the bevelled edges of histiocytosis. North American blastomycosis may give similar lesions and must be considered in regions where it occurs. In the calvarium, TB produces Pott's puffy tumor, a soft-tissue swelling well shown on MR (Fig. 6.28). The skull base is not commonly affected, but the sphenoid bone[34] (Fig. 6.29) and mastoids (Fig. 6.30) may be involved[35]. The facial bones that may be involved are usually the zygoma (Fig. 6.30), maxilla, and angle of the mandible.

Fig. 6.26. Multiple cystic TB in tibia and lower femur.

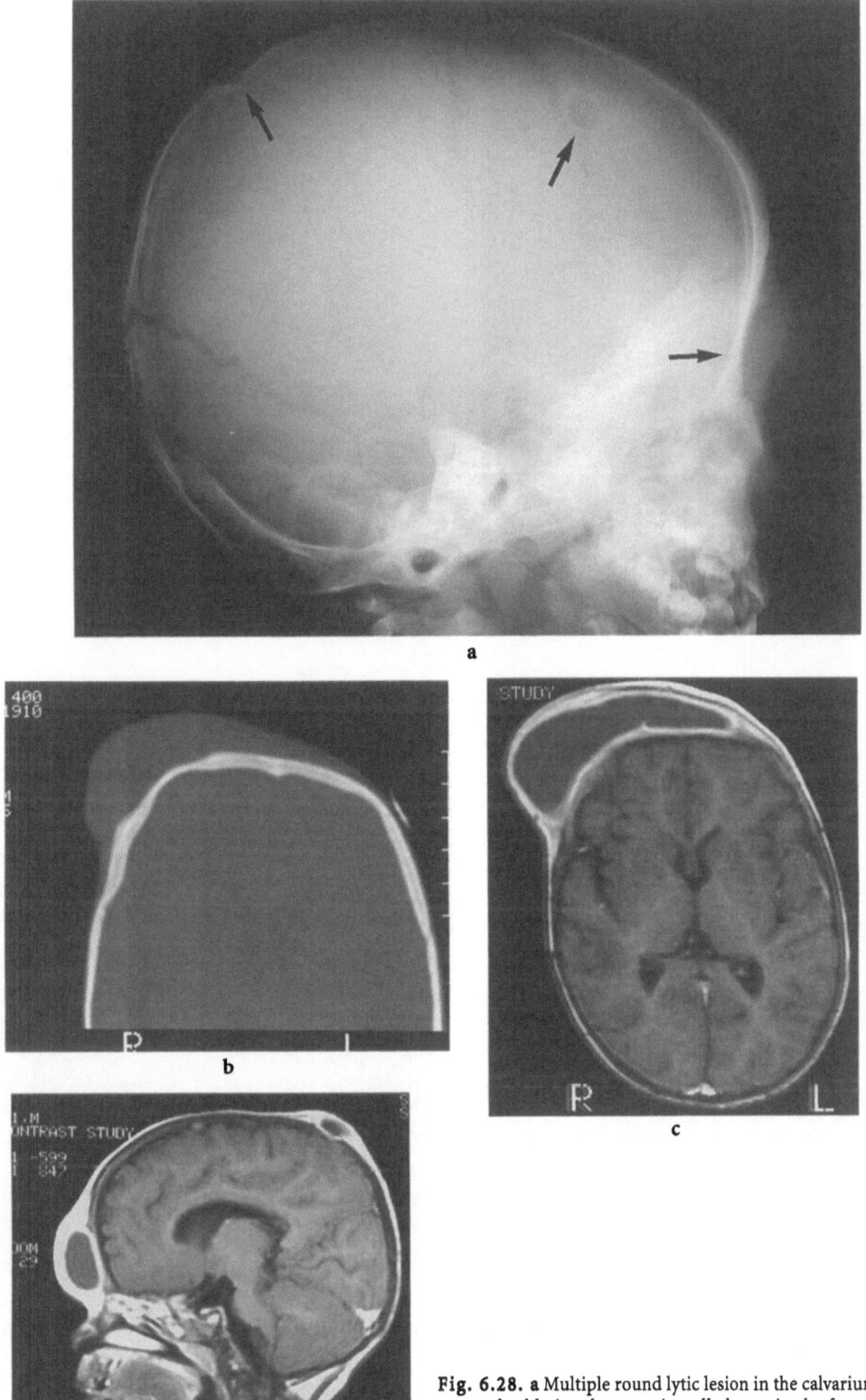

Fig. 6.28. a Multiple round lytic lesion in the calvarium (arrows). The external table involvement is well shown in the frontal lesion. **b** CT showing the frontal lesion involving external table of calvarium. **c,d** Axial and sagittal gadolinium-enhanced MRs demonstrating the calvarial involvement and Pott's puffy tumors.

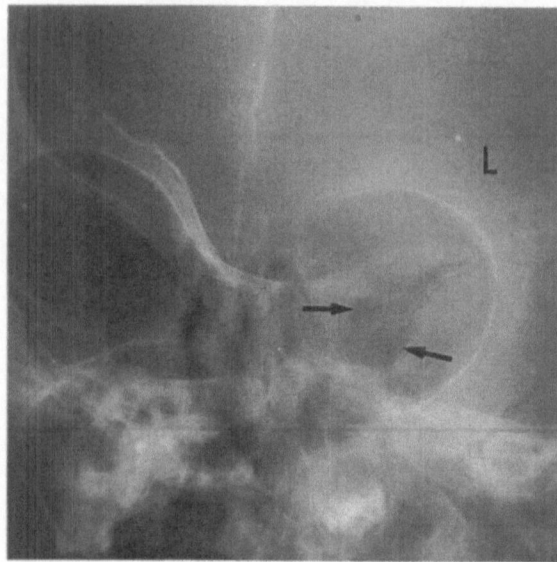

Fig. 6.29. Orbital projection showing destructive changes in left sphenoid bone.

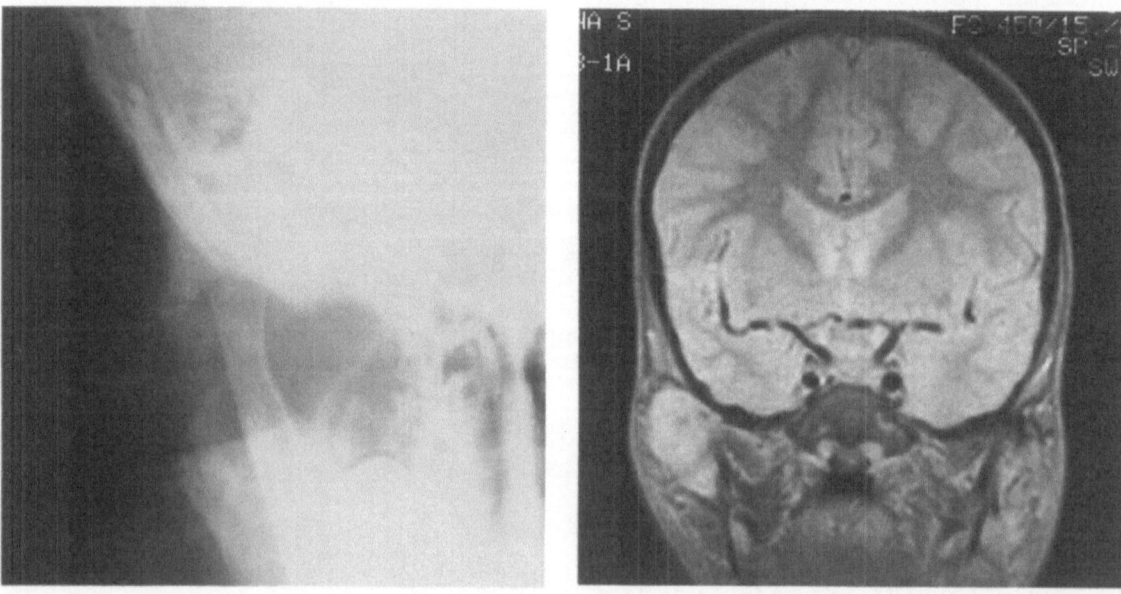

a   b

Fig. 6.30. a Destructive changes in the R zygoma shown by a Townes view. **b** Coronal T2 MR showing destruction of R zygoma and the extent of the soft tissue abscess.

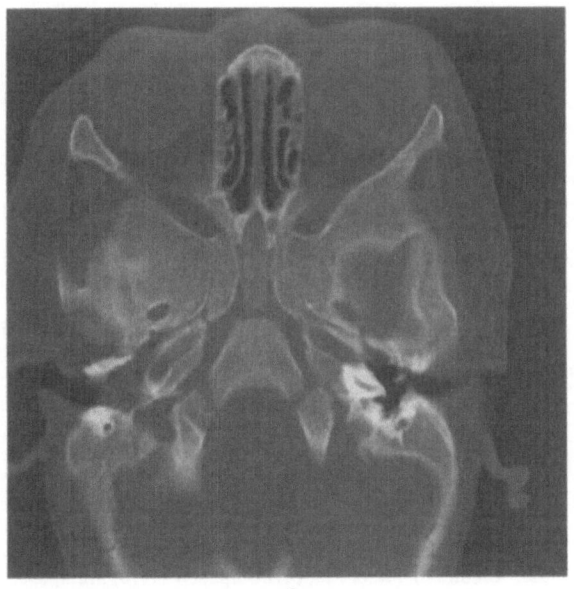

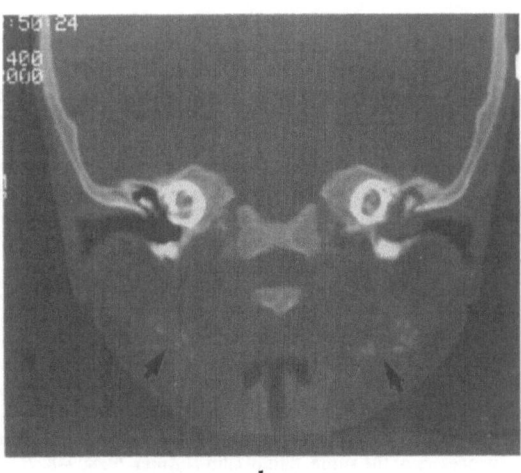

b

a

Fig. 6.31. a Sagittal and **b** coronal CT demonstrating tuberculous destruction of the right inner ear. Calcific glands are seen in the neck (arrow).

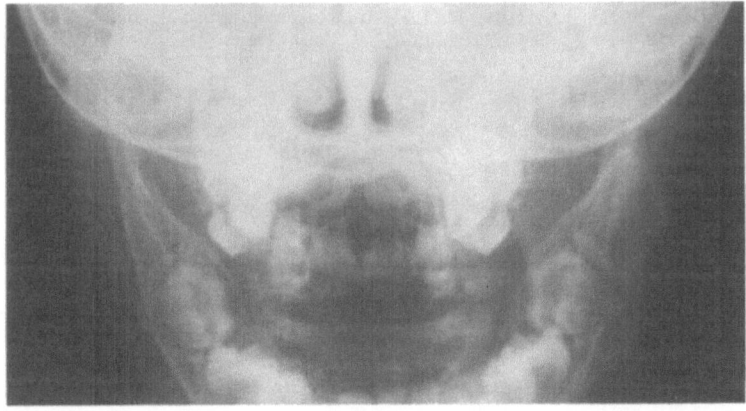

Fig. 6.32. Tuberculous destruction of the angle of the left mandible.

References

1. Shanmugasundaram TK (1987) Bone and joint tuberculosis. Surgery Medical Education (International) Ltd, pp 1060–1066
2. Thijn CJP, Steensma JT (1990) Tuberculosis of the skeleton. Focus on Radiology. Springer Verlag: Heidelberg
3. Allen EH, Cosgrove D, Millard FJ (1978) The radiological changes in infections of the spine and their diagnostic value. Clin Radiol 29: 31–40
4. Goldblatt M, Cremin BJ (1978) Osteo-articular tuberculosis: its presentation in coloured races. Clin Radiol 29: 669–677
5. Chapman M, Murray RO, Stoker DJ (1979) Tuberculosis of the bones and joints. Semin Roentgenol 14: 266–282
6. Reeder MM, Palmer PES (1981) Radiology of Tropical Diseases. Baltimore: Williams & Wilkins, pp 302–346
7. Maritz NGJ, de Villiers JFR, van Casticum QS (1982) Computed tomography in tuberculosis of the spine. Comput Radiol 6: 1–5
8. Gropper GR, Acker JD, Robertson JH (1982) Computed tomography in Pott's disease. Neurosurgery 10: 506–508
9. Hermann G, Mendelson DS, Cohen BA, Train JS (1983) Role of computed tomography in the diagnosis of infectious spondylitis. J Comput Assist Tomog 7: 961–968
10. Whelan MA, Naidich DP, Post JD, Chase NE (1983) Computed tomography of spinal tuberculosis. J Comput Assist Tomogr 7: 25–30
11. La Berge JM, Brant-Zawadski M (1984) Evaluation of Pott's disease with computed tomography. Neuroradiology 26: 429–434
12. Jain R, Sawhney S, Berry M (1993) Computed tomography of vertebral tuberculosis: patterns of bone destruction. Clin Radiol 1993 47: 196–199

13. de Roos A, van Persijn van Meerten EL, Bloem JL, Bluemm RG (1986) MRI of tuberculous spondylitis. AJR 147: 79–82 (Note Vol No misprinted in original article as 146.)

14. Smith AS, Weinstein MA, Mizushima A, Coughlin B, Hayden SP, Lakin MM, Lanziere LF (1989) MR imaging characteristics of tuberculous spondylitis vs vertebral osteomyelitis. AJNR 10: 619–625

15. Hoffman EB, Crosier JH, Cremin BJ (1993) Imaging in children with spinal tuberculosis: a comparison of radiography, computed tomography and magnetic resonance imaging. J Bone Joint Surg [Br] 75B: 233–239

16. Cremin BJ, Jamieson DH, Hoffman EB (1993) CT and MR in the management of advanced spinal tuberculosis. Pediatr Radiol 23: 298–300

17. Hsu LCS, Leong JCY (1984) Tuberculosis of the lower cervical spine (C2 to C7). A report on 40 cases. J Bone Joint Surg [Br] 66B: 1–5

18. Smith AS, Blaser SI (1991) Infectious and inflammatory processes of the spine. Radiol Clin N Amer 29: 809–827

19. Hodgson AR, Wong W, Yau A (1969) Appearances of Tuberculosis of the Spine. Springfield Ill: Charles C Thomas

20. Umerah BC (1977) Radiological patterns of spinal tuberculosis in the African. East Afr Med J 54: 598–605

21. Naim-ur-Rahman (1980) Atypical forms of spinal tuberculosis. J Bone Joint Surg [Br] 62-B: 162–165

22. Campere EL, Garrison M (1936) The correlation of pathological and roentgenological findings in tuberculous and pyogenic infections of the vertebra: the fate of the intervertebral disc. Am Surg 104: 1038–1067

23. Modic MT, Feiglin DH, Piraino DW, Boumphry F, Weinstein MA, Duchesneau PM, Rehm S (1985) Vertebral osteomylitis: assessment using MR. Radiology 157: 157–166

24. Förster A, Pothmann R, Winter K, Baumann-Rath CA (1987) Magnetic resonance imaging in non-specific discitis. Pediatr Radiol 17: 162–163

25. Konstam PG, Bleskovsky A (1962) The ambulant treatment of spinal tuberculosis. Br J Surg 50: 26–38

26. Hodgson AR, Stock FE (1956) Anterior Spinal Fusion: a preliminary on the radical treatment of Pott's disease and Pott's paraplegia. Br J Surg 44: 266–275

27. Controlled trial of short course regimens of chemotherapy in the ambulatory treatment of spinal tuberculosis. (1993) Results of a three year study in Korea. Twelfth report of the Medical Research Council Working Party on tuberculosis of the spine. J Bone Joint Surg [Br] 75B: 240–248

28. Pattisson PRM (1986) Pott's paraplegia: an account of the treatment of 89 conservative patients. Paraplegia 24: 77–91

29. Corr P, Handler L, Davey H (1991) Pott's paraplegia and tuberculous spondylitis: evaluation by magnetic resonance. Neuroradiology 33(suppl): 109–110

30. Kerri O, Martini M (1985) Tuberculosis of the knee. International Orthopaedics (SICOT) 9: 153–157

31. McTammany JR, Moser KM, Houk VN (1963) Disseminated bone tuberculosis. Review of the literature and presentation of an unusual case. Am Rev Respir Dis 37: 889–895

32. Cremin BJ, Fisher RM, Levinsohn MW (1970) Multiple bone tuberculosis in the young. Br J Radiol 43: 638–645

33. Ip M, Tsui E, Wong KL, Jones B, Pung CF, Ngan H (1993) Disseminated skeletal tuberculosis with skull involvement. Tuberc Lung Dis 74: 211–214

34. Witcombe JB, Cremin BJ (1978) Tuberculous erosion of the sphenoid bone. Br J Radiol 51: 347–350

35. Sellars SL (1973) Aural tuberculosis in childhood. S Afr Med J 47: 216–218

7 Clinical Spectrum and Diagnosis of Childhood Tuberculosis

M. Kibel

The recognition of childhood cases of tuberculosis is of particular importance for three reasons.

1. Primary infection is completely asymptomatic in most cases, yet children may harbor a focus which can break down to active disease at any time during life.
2. Progression of disease is most frequent and dangerous in young children and if not diagnosed and treated, may lead to death or chronic disablement.
3. Every newly infected child represents recent transmission from an infectious source, and failure of our ability to control tuberculosis[1].

M. tuberculosis is almost always acquired by inhalation from an infectious person. Rarely, it may enter the body through the oro-pharynx, throat, eye or skin. A variety of other mycobacteria also cause human disease but with a generally milder clinical spectrum. *M. bovis*, the cause of tuberculosis in cattle, occurs through the ingestion of infected milk, infection thus occurring via the organs of the gastro-intestinal tract and draining lymph nodes. Today, tuberculosis of the gastro-intestinal tract is generally caused by human tuberculosis, and not by the bovine variety.

The Natural History

Pulmonary tuberculosis in childhood has many faces. There is a full spectrum of clinical severity, ranging from totally silent infection to acute and rampant disease. The reasons for this wide sweep of clinical effects lie in the complex double immune response induced by tuberculous infection. On the one hand, there is protective cellular immunity which restricts the multiplication of mycobacteria. On the other, there is the delayed hypersensitivity response with induced inflammation and necrosis of tissue[2]. During chemotherapy the development of delayed hypersensitivity may result in unexpected clinical changes in the child[3].

In the majority of cases primary infection passes unnoticed. Only if a tuberculin test is performed will it be realized that infection has taken place. Careful observation may detect the occurrence of transient fever or malaise[4].

Even without recognition and treatment, healing occurs in most cases. The primary complex may be microscopic, and completely eliminated. Larger lesions are walled off by fibrosis and calcification may ensue. The lymph node component takes longer to regress than the pulmonary focus. Organisms may, however, remain dormant within macrophages, with a life-long potential for endogenous reactivation should the immune system be depressed for any reason.

The first 6 months following infection is a period of great danger. It is during this period that progression of the primary focus and the development of disseminated forms of TB are particularly likely to develop. Pleural effusions tend to occur 3–6 months after initial infection. Skeletal TB generally shows itself later, after 1–2 years. Renal TB only rarely presents in the childhood years[5,6].

Factors Leading to the Progression of the Primary Complex

A number of factors affect the child's response to the initial infection. Age is of paramount importance. Children under 5 years old, and especially those under 1 year, are able to mount far less resistance to the organism and dissemination is especially common. Up to 43% of infected infants under 1 year of age will have radiological evidence of tuberculous disease, compared with 24% of children aged 1–5 years, and 15% of 11–15-year-olds[7]. Over-crowding leads to more frequent exposure, and poor ventilation to greater concentrations of bacilli. A child who is malnourished or suffering from some other infection or infestation is more likely to acquire overt disease and more likely to develop the severe forms. There is less risk of progressive primary disease in later childhood. The adolescent years again represent a high risk period, but now for the development of adult-type pulmonary tuberculosis, characterized immunologically by a necrotizing response and radiologically by the development of cavitation. Females are 2–6 times more susceptible to disease during this period, and an as yet unidentified endocrinological influence is usually held responsible for these events[8].

Poor nutrition and dietary deficiencies certainly play an important role in lowering resistance to the spread of the bacilli. Conversely, tuberculous infection itself may tip a child with borderline nutrition into a decompensated state of marasmus or kwashiorkor, both from the stress of the infection and the presence of abdominal tuberculosis, which often results in a protein-losing enteropathy.

Any infection which lowers general resistance during the period of early primary TB may result in progression of the disease. Measles and whooping cough are particularly dangerous in this respect. HIV infection must now rank as the most important inducer and propagator of frank tuberculous disease[9]. Initial evidence seems to indicate that the relationship between HIV infection/AIDS and tuberculosis may be just as ominous in children as in adults[10].

Clinical Spectrum of Progressive Primary Disease

Progression of the primary complex causes illness in the child, but symptoms and signs are subtle and still often go unrecognized. Mild intermittent fever and slight cough both persisting for some weeks are frequent, or the child may simply seem unwell and below par. Loss of weight or flagging weight gain may be experienced. TB should always be suspected in underweight infants or children, particularly those who fail to show catch-up on full dietary replacement.

Clinical examination of the chest will generally reveal no positive findings at this stage. An area of opacification in the lung together with a prominent hilum or broadened mediastinal shadow may or may not be clearly definable on chest X-ray. Disease of this order may still resolve spontaneously without the diagnosis being made or effective treatment instituted. Fibrous scarring and calcification will then appear in the lung and/or lymph nodes after about a year as a long-lasting record of the disease. There is, however, a grave risk of progression and dissemination without treatment.

Once tuberculous infection has gained entry into the hilar nodes, extension can occur not only to other lymph nodes in the chest but also to those far distant from the primary infection, in the neck, axilla or abdomen.

As nodes enlarge and become adherent to each other a large caseating mass may develop in one or both hila or in the upper or lower mediastinum. The child is generally symptomatic, with fever, loss of weight, cough or other respiratory symptoms, but any or all of these may be inconspicuous or absent.

When glands become adherent to the bronchi above and below the carina, or to the trachea, the bronchial tree itself becomes involved in the inflammatory process and lymphobronchial disease ensues. Cough becomes troublesome and persistent. Inspiratory stridor and brassy cough are characteristic features of enlarged paratracheal glands. Wheezing results from pressure of glands around the carina and major bronchi. If only one bronchus is involved wheezing may be confined to one lung only, but generalized wheezing is more common. The lungs are hyper-resonant to percussion due to generalized air trapping.

Inflammation from adherent tuberculous glands may spread further throughout the full thickness of the bronchial wall, resulting in granulations within the bronchial lumen itself. The following clinical syndromes can result from lymphobronchial disease:

1. *Over-inflated Lungs*. Partial obstruction of the bronchus results in air gaining entry into the lung on inspiration but total blockage on expiration – a "ball valve" effect leading to lobar emphysema. The acute distress can be relieved with oxygen, and nebulized salbutamol and oral corticosteroids are beneficial. Further diagnostic evaluation and management in hospital is generally indicated.

2. *Segmental Lesion*. Complete obstruction of a bronchus results in atelectasis of that portion of lung distal to the obstruction, usually the right middle or right lower lobe or a segment thereof. Caseating material may enter the lung, resulting in spread of tuberculous disease to that segment

or lobe, or the collapsed area may be otherwise healthy but become secondarily infected. In many cases re-expansion or clearing occurs after about 3–6 months of anti-tuberculous treatment[11]. In a substantial proportion re-expansion never occurs and the end result is a permanently damaged bronchiectatic lobe following years of recurrent secondary infection[12].

3. *Tuberculous bronchopneumonia*. Massive extrusion of caseating material from glands into the bronchial tree results in wide-spread dissemination of infection throughout both lungs. This picture may ensue quite suddenly with dramatic worsening in the child's condition, with fever, respiratory difficulty, wide-spread crackles on auscultation, and rapid deterioration unless effective treatment is instituted.

4. *Rarer manifestations*. Three rarer manifestations should be mentioned:

i. Entrapment of the phrenic nerve in caseating tissue can result in paralysis of the diaphragm.

ii. Lymphatic obstruction and/or damage to one of the lymphatic ducts sometimes results in massive chylothorax with or without ascites.

iii. Tuberculous erosion through the full thickness of the bronchial wall or esophagus can result in the passage of air, fluid or food into the pleural cavity. Pneumothorax and empyema and bronchopleural or bronchoesphageal fistulae are the consequence of such advanced disease and present complex management problems[13].

Tuberculous Pneumonia

The tuberculous process spreads rapidly throughout a segment or entire lobe. Both clinically and radiologically the picture may be difficult or impossible to distinguish from that of simple bacterial pneumonia. The illness should be treated with antibiotics on the basis of a straight-forward pneumonia while at the same time investigations for tuberculosis should be instituted. Given the insidious nature of primary tuberculosis it is not surprising that many children with primary tuberculosis and its complications are fortuitously diagnosed during the course of investigation of other intercurrent illnesses.

Tuberculosis of the Pleura

The sudden accumulation of pleural fluid is largely a hypersensitivity phenomenon induced by a primary focus contiguous to the pleura. Despite the dramatic X-ray appearances, the illness is not necessarily severe or progressive. The child complains of dull chest pain or breathlessness associated with cough but is otherwise relatively well. Hospitalization is required, as the effusion should always be aspirated for diagnostic purposes, examined for organisms and cultured to exclude pyogenic causes. Adenosine deaminase (ADA) is raised (above 35 units) and this test is of value in distinguishing TB from other causes of pleural effusion. The tuberculin reaction is usually strongly reactive. Children with a pleural effusion tend to be above the age of 5 years, older than those with the forms of disease already described. When pleural involvement occurs in younger children it is more often associated with extensive pulmonary disease. There is thickening and caseation of the pleura with only minimal amounts of encysted fluid. The tuberculin test is often negative or only slightly reactive.

Spontaneous pneumothorax is a well-recognized complication of pleural TB.

Blood-Spread Dissemination

Miliary tuberculosis results from massive spread of mycobacteria into the bloodstream. Although the appearances in the lungs are characteristic, the tiny granulomata are distributed widely throughout the body. It is commonest in young infants when resistance to infection is impaired, but can occur at any age. The onset may be abrupt with high fever and severe illness, or insidious with surprisingly little general disturbance[14]. Fever and malaise may precede the appearance of radiological changes by several days. Such infants almost always show evidence of weight loss, enlargement of liver and spleen or generalized lymphadenopathy. Careful ophthalmoscopic examination of the retina may show choroid tubercles – round white to yellow cotton-wool-like lesions – situated near the retinal vessels. Lumbar puncture will yield abnormal CSF, in about 25% of cases indicative of early tuberculous meningitis. If there has been erosion into a pulmonary arteriole, miliary spread may be confined to the lungs or even to a single lung, so that liver and splenic enlargement are not noted.

In some individuals hematogenous dissemination may be cryptogenic, manifesting only with fever and cachexia[15]. At the other end of the spectrum, individual foci of dissemination can show themselves sporadically in bone, soft tissues, or any other organ, over many months or years[16].

Lymphadenitis

Tuberculous lymph glands are most commonly encountered in the neck, but may also be present in the axillae or groins. Characteristically, there is painless enlargement of a group of nodes in the supraclavicular region, posterior, or anterior cervical lymph chains. The nodes coelesce as they caseate and become adherent to skin, forming subcutaneous cold abscesses. Eventually, over the course of 6–12 months discharging fistulae are formed[17].

TB cervical lymphadenitis is most commonly due to extension up the lymphatic system from nodes in the mediastinum. A few cases may be due to primary tuberculous infection in the oral cavity or tonsils and caused by human or bovine disease. In countries with low prevalence of tuberculosis, mycobacteria other than tubercle are common causes of lymphadenitis but for some reason seem to be rare in higher prevalence settings[18].

Where fluctuation or frank fistulae are present, material can readily be obtained by aspiration for microscopy culture and sensitivity testing. When this is not the case biopsy of enlarged nodes is mandatory, both to establish the diagnosis of mycobacterial infection and to obtain material for culture and sensitivity.

Manifestations of Hypersensitivity

A minority of children develop clinical manifestations of hypersensitivity to tubercular protein.

Phlyctenular conjunctivitis: one or more tiny raised nodules at the junction of the corneal and palpebral conjunctiva, with surrounding conjunctival injection, and associated with considerable discomfort and photophobia.

Erythema nodosum: tender red, or bruise-like areas of induration over both lower legs, associated with pain in the ankles, and sometimes in other joints. Poncet's arthritis: an acute arthropathy of the finger joints, and/or one or more large joints.

The Tuberculin Skin Test

The cellular immune response is assessed by the tuberculin skin test. This is a delayed hypersensitivity reaction and skin reactivity indicates that infection with mycobacteria has occurred. A positive tuberculin skin test is the hallmark of the primary infection. Few tests in medical practise are as widely used yet as misunderstood. Only the tubercle bacillus induces a strong skin reaction, but BCG and other mycobacteria cause lesser skin responses which result in confusion in interpretation. To use it effectively one must be familiar with its limitations and variations[1].

The most accurate method of tuberculin testing is the Mantoux test. This is carried out by injecting 0.1-ml diluted tuberculin intradermally using a very small gauge (size 27) needle. A suitable dose is 5 tuberculin units (TU) of purified protein derivative (PPD). In children it is particularly difficult to insert the needle accurately and care must be taken to see that a wheal appears in the skin as the fluid is injected. If the injection is too deep a false negative result may be obtained. The test is quantitative, and is read as the transverse diameter of induration present at 48–72 h. It is positive if there is an area of induration (not only color alteration) greater than 10 mm in diameter. A transverse induration of 15 mm and greater indicates infection with *M. tuberculosis*, even if BCG has been given. An induration of 10 mm and greater indicates infection with *M. tuberculosis* if BCG has not been given. Induration of from 5 to 9 mm may indicate infection with *M. tuberculosis* but can also result from BCG immunization or contact with a typical mycobacterium.

Multiple puncture tests are more convenient and easier to administer and in practise they are widely used in clinic situations. It must be realized, however, that these are only qualitative screening tests. The older Heaf Test has generally been superseded. Several commercial disposable multiple puncture kits are available and are particularly useful when only occasional tuberculin tests are required.

In some, the antigen is dried on the prongs and in others it is liquid. One example is the Tine Test. It consists of a disposable thimble with 4 sharp tines, the tips of which are coated with dried PPD. The test is read after 3–7 days using the following criteria: Positive: confluence of two or more papules with or without vesication.

Negative or doubtful: any lesser reaction. If suspicion of TB is high, retest with Mantoux within 1 week.

The tuberculin test is an essential part of the diagnosis of childhood tuberculosis. The test is highly reliable if properly performed with active tuberculin and properly-maintained equipment. Anergy, resulting in a negative test, occurs from certain well-defined causes, namely very severe infection with *M. tuberculosis*, serious malnutrition, severe viral infections or any condition that suppresses the immune system. As stated earlier, measles is an important infection which induces this anergy which may persist for up to 2 months after the infection. Similar, though less prolonged, suppression occurs following measles vaccination. Other infections which cause temporary suppression of the tuberculin reaction include rubella, scarlet fever, pertussis, infectious mononucleosis, influenza and malaria.

Infection with HIV is an important consideration as a cause of a suppressed immune response to mycobacteria. If treatment for tuberculosis is started on the assumption that anergy is present, the test must be repeated after a month, when the majority of these factors will have been corrected, to confirm the diagnosis.

A positive reaction indicates that infection with tubercle bacilli has occurred. It does not necessarily mean that active disease is present. A negative reaction certainly does not rule out the presence of active disease[19].

Bacteriological Confirmation of Tuberculosis in Childhood

The "gold standard" of diagnosis is identification of mycobacteria on microscopy and/or culture. Whereas the diagnosis of active tuberculosis in adults is mainly bacteriologic, this is unfortunately the exception rather than the rule in children. The reasons are threefold: (a) organisms are not generally present in great numbers in childhood TB as they are in adult-type cavitatory disease, and the release of organisms from the lung parenchyma into the bronchial tree is a transitory or a late phenomenon; (b) young children are unable to produce sputum and this must be obtained by aspirating swallowed sputum from the stomach; (c) examination of gastric fluid is subject to interpretative errors: false positives are frequent on direct microscopic examination, whereas successful culture requires correct handling of specimens, with adjustment of the acid pH as soon as they are obtained. It is not surprising therefore that reports on the bacteriological yield in childhood TB vary widely, but overall are no higher than 25%[20]. Nevertheless, where resources are available, every attempt should be made to identify the organism both in order to reach a firm diagnosis and to establish the drug sensitivity profile. If possible, 3 early morning samples should be obtained by gastric aspiration.

Less usually, material is obtained by bronchoscopy, but the yield has been reported to be no better than by gastric aspiration[21].

Diagnosis

The diagnosis of TB generally rests on a consideration of:

1. history of contact with an infectious case
2. symptoms and signs
3. the tuberculin test
4. the radiological appearances.

History of Contact with an Infectious Case

The importance of an adequate history of exposure cannot be over-emphasized. Of particular significance are close contacts – affected parents or affected individuals who sleep in the same room as the child. It is obviously also crucially important to rule out TB in all contacts of newly diagnosed cases. A great responsibility rests on the provider of primary health care. It is at this point of first contact that the disease may be recognized and investigated further.

Symptoms

Suspicion of tuberculosis is halfway to diagnosis. Health professionals must be sensitized to the suggestive symptoms – loss of weight and lassitude, cough, wheeze or stridor which have lasted for more than 2–3 weeks, or failure to rehabilitate or catch-up in severe malnutrition.

Radiology

While the chest X-ray (CXR) remains one of the main pillars of diagnosis, it must be emphasized that in the clinical situations where most cases are diagnosed, routine CXRs may be confusing or unhelpful. This is because

1. they are of poor quality technically
2. the Ghon lesion is too small to be visualized by routine methods
3. nodes may be obscured in the mediastinal shadow.

Other Investigations

Histology. Biopsy of liver, bone marrow, pleura or superficial lymph node may assist in the diagnosis. Material must be sent for both histology and culture.

Serology. ELISA antigen capture and antibody detection techniques are cheap and rapid serogical tests. They have not as yet been introduced for general use, as both sensitivity and specificity vary in different hands, but they offer great promise as an aid in cases of diagnostic uncertainty and particularly in TB meningitis[22].

DNA Probes. The practicality of identifying mycobacterial-specific genetic material by PCR has been demonstrated by many groups. Unfortunately, very few laboratories can yet offer this method for routine use.

Problems in Diagnosis

The diagnosis of tuberculosis in childhood is complicated by the spectrum of infection and disease which is encountered, and which, depending upon the age of the child and the severity of illness, might be considered as requiring therapy, despite relatively flimsy evidence. Applying the diagnostic standards of the American Thoracic Society[23], the following groups can be identified:

1. Children in close contact with an adult case of pulmonary tuberculosis, but with a negative tuberculin test, and no radiological or clinical signs of disease. Depending partly on age, such children are considered to be at considerable risk of developing disease. Children in this category should be placed on prophylactic therapy and re-evaluated after 2–3 months. If the tuberculin test remains negative, and no signs of disease are encountered, treatment can be stopped at this point, and the child vaccinated with BCG.

2. Children with a significantly positive tuberculin test. These children are considered to be at a preclinical stage of infection with *M. tuberculosis*. Particularly in the very young it can be presumed that this infection is recent and thus still active, and that there is a significant risk of disease. Such children should be placed on at least 6 months of isoniazid. This approach is supported by the frequency with which cultures of *M. tuberculosis* can be obtained from such apparently normal children[24,25].

3. Tuberculosis is considered to be clinically active in those with "clinical and/or radiographic evidence" of current tuberculosis. The tuberculin test is generally (but by no means invariably) significantly positive. A culture of *M. tuberculosis* confirms the diagnosis, but this is obtained in a minority of cases in children.

4. Tuberculosis, not clinically active, includes those with a history of previous tuberculosis, or abnormal, but stable radiographic findings in the presence of a positive tuberculin test and no other evidence of current active disease.

5. Suspected tuberculosis. Particularly in developing communities, this group will include many children with persistent respiratory symptoms or signs, loss of weight or failure to gain in weight or failure to recover from an intercurrent illness. Taking into consideration factors such as age, severity of illness, and contact with an adult case of pulmonary TB (PTB), such children will often be treated for tuberculosis until more diagnostic clarity is obtained.

The diagnosis of TB in childhood is therefore often not an easy matter and is influenced by a history of contact with an adult, a suspicious-looking CXR or failure to gain adequately in weight. Unfortunately, in developing countries where tuberculosis is often endemic, many children who do not have tuberculosis will have a history of close contact with an adult case of PTB. Similarly, although many children being treated for tuberculosis will have a recent loss of weight or failure to thrive, many children with obvious radiological abnormalities will in fact be gaining adequately in weight[26].

Tuberculosis and Human Immunodeficiency Virus Infection

Lowered immuno-defences against mycobacterial infections occur very early in HIV infection, and TB is frequently the first manifestation of this illness in adults. The recent world-wide increase in tuberculosis is influenced by the burgeoning population of HIV-positive individuals. In sub-Saharan Africa, assuming a 2% annual risk of tuberculosis infection, a 60% tuberculosis infection prevalence, and a 20% HIV prevalence, a tenfold increase in smear-positive tuberculosis rates in adults can be predicted. In children, this could potentially lead to rates of 2500 cases/100,000 amongst children under 15 years of age[27].

About 80% of HIV-positive children are infected by their mothers, mostly while in utero. Infection can also result from breast feeding, from receiving blood, or blood products, and through sexual abuse. The course of the illness is more rapid in the very young, where impairment of immunocompetence results in frequent and recurrent infections due to a wide range of common pathogens. Non-specific symptoms and signs of HIV disease include low birth weight, failure to thrive, recurrent respiratory infections, oral thrush, recurrent diarrhoea, unexplained fever, chronic dermatitis, persistent lymphadenopathy, hepatosplenomegaly, anemia and thrombocytopenia[28]. The difficulties in diagnosing TB in children alluded to earlier are greatly magnified in the HIV-positive child. Not only may TB be atypical in its presentation, but it must also be distinguished from a range of other opportunistic respiratory pathogens – *Pneumocystis carinii, Cytomegalovirus, Candida albicans*, and other fungi, as well as other mycobacteria. Lymphoid interstitial pneumonitis, possibly due to the HIV virus itself, must also be excluded. TB may also present in highly unusual forms in HIV-infected adolescents. Further elaboration on this complex subject is beyond the scope of this chapter.

References

1. Starke JR, Jacobs RF, Jereb J (1992). Resurgence of tuberculosis in children. J Pediat 120: 839–855
2. Grange J (1994). Modern concepts of immunity in tuberculosis. In: Donald PR, Van de Wal BW (eds) Tuberculosis 1992. University of Stellenbosch, Stellenbosch pp 40–50
3. Lenzini L, Tottoli P, Rottoli L (1977). The spectrum of human tuberculosis. Clin Exp Immunol 27: 230–7
4. Wallgren A (1935). Primary pulmonary tuberculosis in childhood. Am J Dis Child 5: 1105–1136
5. Wallgren A (1948). The time-table of tuberculosis. Tubercle 29: 245–251

6. Lincoln EM (1950). Course and prognosis of tuberculosis in children. Am J Med 9: 623–632
7. Miller FJW, Seale RME, Taylor MD (1982). Tuberculosis in Children
8. Smith MHD (1967). Tuberculosis in adolescents: characteristics, recognition, management. Clin Pediatr 6: 9–15
9. Barnes PF, Block AB, Davidson PT, Snider DE Jr. (1991). Tuberculosis in patients with human immunodeficiency virus infection. N Eng J Med 324: 1644–50
10. Chintu C, Bhat G, Luo C, Ravigliont M, Diwan V, Dupont HL, Zumla A (1993). Seroprevalence of human immunodeficiency virus type 1 infection in Zambian children with tuberculosis. Pediatr Infect Dis J 12: 499–504
11. Morrison JB (1973). Natural history of segmental lesions in primary pulmonary tuberculosis. Arch Dis Child 48: 90–98
12. Lincoln EM, Harris LC, Bovornkitti S, Carretero RW (1958) Endobronchial tuberculosis in children. Am Rev Tuberc 77: 39–61
13. Shope RE, Petersdorf RG (1959) Mediastinal tuberculosis manifested by pericarditis, osteochondritis, and broncho esophageal fistula. Am Rev TB 79: 238–243
14. Illingworth RS (1956) Miliary and meningeal tuberculosis. Difficulties in diagnosis. Lancet 271: 646–649
15. Emery JL, Lorber J (1950). Radiological and pathological correlation of miliary tuberculosis of the lungs in children. Br Med J 2: 702–704
16. Debre R (1952). Miliary tuberculosis in children. Lancet 2: 545–549
17. Miller FJW, Cashman JM (1955). The natural history of peripheral tuberculous lymphadenitis associated with a visible primary focus. Lancet 1: 1286–1289
18. Margileth AM, Chandra R, Altman RP (1984). Chronic lymphadenopathy due to mycobacterial infection. Am J Dis Child 138: 917–922
19. Steiner P, Rao M, Victoria MS, Jabbar H, Steiner M (1980). Persistently negative tuberculin reactions. Am J Dis Child 134: 747–750
20. Starke JR, Taylor-Watts KT (1989). Tuberculosis in the pediatic population of Houston, Texas. Pediatrics 84: 28–35
21. de Blic J, Azevedo I, Burrel CP, Le Bourgeois M, Lallemand D, Scheinmann P (1991). The value of flexible bronchoscopy in childhood pulmonary tuberculosis. Chest 100: 688–92
22. Hussey G, Kibel MA, Dempster W (1991). The serodiagnosis of tuberculosis in children: an evaluation of an ELISA test using IgG antibodies to M.tuberculosis, strain H37 RV. Ann Trop Paediatr 11: 113–118
23. Bass JB, Farer LS, Hopewell PC, Jacobs RF, Snider DE (1990). Diagnostic standards and classification of tuberculosis. Am Rev Respir Dis 42: 725–735
24. Toppet M, Malfroot A, Hofman B, Casmir G, Contraine F, Dab I (1991). Tuberculosis in children: a 13 year follow up of 1714 patients in a Belgian home care centre. Europ J Pediatr 150: 331–335
25. Fox TG (1977). Occult tuberculous infection in children. Tubercle 58: 91–96
26. Hennink MJ, Skibbe A, Donald PR (1988). Failure to gain in weight prior to the diagnosis of pulmonary tuberculosis. J Trop Pediatr 34: 108–109
27. Schulzer M. Fitzgerald JM, Enarson DA, Grzybowski S (1992). An estimate of the future size of the tuberculosis problem in sub-Saharan Africa resulting from HIV infection. Tubercle Lung Dis 73: 52–58
28. Burroughs MH, Edelson PJ (1991). Medical care of the HIV-infected child. Pediatr Clin North Am 38: 45–67

8 Drug Treatment and Resistance

P.R. Donald

The treatment of tuberculosis in childhood has in the past rested upon the principles developed for, and applied to, the treatment of adult tuberculosis. Children have thus been considered as "therapeutic orphans" and treated empirically with regimens similar to those used in adults, but with some adjustment of dosages[1].

Increased knowledge of the actions of antituberculosis medications and an appreciation of the mycobacterial populations likely to be present in different types of lesions has led to the more rational use of anti-tuberculosis drugs in childhood and several groups have now described the follow-up of children treated with short course regimens and confirmed their applicability to children.

Special Mycobacterial Populations

Mycobacteria can be considered to exist in tuberculosis lesions in different populations classified according to their metabolic activity[2]. Within the cavities often associated with "adult type" tuberculosis, but infrequent in childhood, there is a large population of metabolically active, rapidly dividing mycobacteria. These organisms are particularly susceptible to the actions of isoniazid and, to a lesser extent, rifampicin and streptomycin. The size of this population is estimated to be in the region of 10^8 organisms. Two considerably smaller populations each consisting of 10^4–10^5 organisms are found within the relatively unfavorable conditions that exist in solid caseous tissue and within macrophages. Many of these organisms are thought to be only intermittently active; rifampicin is particularly valuable in this situation, given the speed with which it starts to act[3,4]. Pyrazinamide has a negligible effect upon the rapidly dividing organisms within cavities and acts mainly against those organisms which lie within the acid environment of the macrophage. It has thus an important role in sterilizing tuberculous lesions and appears to fulfil this role within the first 2 months of therapy.

The small fourth population of organisms lies dormant within the macrophage; they are probably not affected by any anti-tuberculosis drug while metabolically inactive. A number of clinical studies in adults have confirmed that isoniazid and rifampicin given for 6 months and pyrazinamide given for the first 2 months of therapy will cure from 96% to 99% of adult patients with initially fully drug-sensitive organisms.

The combination of these three valuable drugs isoniazid, rifampicin and pyrazinamide has revolutionized the treatment of tuberculosis and made possible regimens of 6–months' duration now usually referred to as short course chemotherapy.

Prevention of Drug Resistance

It became apparent shortly after streptomycin became available for the treatment of tuberculosis that resistance to streptomycin developed fairly rapidly in a significant proportion of patients. With the addition of other medications such as isoniazid and para-amino salicylic acid (PAS) to the treatment regimen it was realized that the development of resistance could be prevented by combination therapy. It is now known that any population of mycobacteria will harbor a small number of drug-resistant mutants[5] and that the success of a drug in preventing the development of resistance will depend on its ability to inhibit mycobacteria in all of the patient's lesions throughout treatment[3]. The most effective drugs for preventing the development of resistance to other drugs when used in combination therapy are considered to be isoniazid and rifampicin. Pyrazinamide, PAS and thiacetazone are less successful.

In summary, then, short-course chemotherapy in adult forms of pulmonary tuberculosis can be considered to have 3 aims which are fulfilled during 2 phases of treatment.

1. The rapid elimination of the majority of actively dividing mycobacteria to reduce and control the amount of damage to the patient's lungs and to eliminate the danger of infection amongst close contacts. The most effective agent in this phase of bactericidal action is isoniazid and up to 90% of the mycobacterial population is killed within days of starting chemotherapy.

2. The prevention of the development of a population of drug-resistant mycobacteria by the use of drug combinations. The low incidence with which mutations occur makes it unlikely that resistance to two or more drugs will arise in the same organism de novo. The most effective drugs for this purpose should constantly inhibit bacterial proliferation in all of a patient's tuberculous lesions.

3. The sterilization of all of the patient's lesions to prevent relapse when treatment is completed. Semi-dormant, intermittently active, mycobacteria may survive the action of isoniazid. Those that are extracellular are thought to be killed mainly by the relatively rapid onset of action of rifampicin while those that are intracellular are killed by pyrazinamide and rifampicin.

The Phases of Treatment

During the 2-month *initial phase* of treatment the killing of the bulk of the bacillary population occurs, particularly under the influence of isoniazid. It is also during this period that pyrazinamide appears to achieve its maximum effect. This is followed by a 4-month *continuation phase* during which the surviving mycobacteria are eliminated by isoniazid and in particular by rifampicin.

Thus modern short-course chemotherapy of adult pulmonary tuberculosis in areas where drug resistance is not a problem will consist of isoniazid and rifampicin given for 6 months augmented by pyrazinamide for the first 2 months of treatment.

Applicability of the Principles of Short-Course Treatment to Childhood Tuberculosis

In childhood tuberculosis it seems probable that relatively small numbers of semi-dormant or dormant organisms will be found within the caseous tissue of the primary focus or the regional lymph nodes and within macrophages. Exceptions would be those children with cavitating lung lesions and extensive lobar or bronchopneumonic disease or disseminated miliary tuberculosis. The relatively small number of bacilli present in most children also implies that there will usually be a low risk of resistant mutants arising[6].

In view of the satisfactory experience of short-course chemotherapy in adults with far more extensive disease than is usually seen in children there was little doubt amongst clinicians that 6 months of anti-tuberculosis therapy should be more than adequate for children amongst whom it is notoriously difficult to culture *M. tuberculosis* from any source and even more difficult to find acid-fast bacilli on microscopy of sputum or gastric aspirate. In recent years several groups have published their experience with short-course chemotherapy in children and have commented upon the satisfactory results achieved [7,8,9].

Duration Of Therapy

Most forms of pediatric tuberculosis can be compared to radiologically positive, but sputum-microscopy and culture negative, adult pulmonary tuberculosis with limited parenchymal involvement. It is now clear that treatment of this form of adult pulmonary tuberculosis for 4 months with rifampicin and isoniazid and with pyrazinamide for the initial 2 months yields very low relapse rates[10,11]. As the bacillary populations present in these patients are probably similar to those in children it is now suggested by the World Health Organization that this group of children should be treated in similar fashion[12]. The longer, more conventional 6-month regimen should be used in those children with more extensive parenchymal involvement or with extrapulmonary tuberculosis.

Patient Adherence to the Prescribed Regimen

It has been the unhappy experience of tuberculosis control programmes throughout the world that a substantial proportion of patients do not adhere to the prescribed regimens. This failure of compliance may be compounded by poor administration of control programmes[13]. This may lead not only to dire consequences for patients and their families, but also to the development of drug resistance and consequently a serious threat to the tuberculosis control programme and the use of short-course chemotherapy[14]. This threat has been exacerbated by the rise in AIDS, the association of AIDS and HIV infection and tuberculosis, and the fact that those populations and sub-populations which are susceptible to HIV infection and AIDS are precisely those groups which have a high incidence of tuberculosis[15]. This threat to the patient and to the control programme can best be prevented by insistence upon supervised therapy whenever possible. This means that all therapy should be seen to be taken by someone other than the patient. Such a supervisor need not be a health worker, but should be acceptable to the patient as a supervisor.

Because most children with tuberculosis have relatively small bacillary populations, the danger of the development of drug resistance as a result of failure of compliance is not as great as in adults. Insistence upon supervized therapy for children should thus be balanced by the operational needs of the tuberculosis control programme in a particular area.

Chemoprophylaxis

It is well established that the development of tuberculous disease in infected persons can be prevented by the use of isoniazid taken for at least 6 months[16]. In adults the efficacy of chemoprophylaxis must be balanced by the possibility of hepatic toxicity, which may be associated with the use of isoniazid. In children, however, hepatotoxicity is an uncommon problem and the decision to institute chemoprophylaxis is an operational one influenced by clinical and epidemiological considerations.

Children with the highest risk of developing serious forms of tuberculosis are young children, especially those less than 2 years of age[17] and those in contact with adults who are excreting sputum which is positive on microscopy for acid-fast bacilli[18]. The

risk of developing disease following infection is particularly high during the first 2 years after infection[19]. If such individuals can be identified by tuberculin testing or a history of exposure, they will undoubtedly benefit from chemoprophylaxis. Children less than 5 years of age who have a significantly positive tuberculin test can also be assumed to have been recently infected.

The persistence and diligence with which chemoprophylaxis should be pursued will again depend upon the epidemiological situation in the area concerned. In an area of low incidence of tuberculosis and sufficient community resources it may be possible to pursue the ideal of chemoprophylaxis of every tuberculin-positive individual with the aim of ultimately eliminating tuberculosis. More often, however, the tuberculosis control services will be hard pressed to diagnose and manage all the cases of adult pulmonary tuberculosis occurring within a particular area and will have to accord a much lower priority to chemoprophylaxis. A compromise in this respect might be to insist on supervised chemoprophylaxis for the very young contacts of pulmonary tuberculosis patients with smear positive sputum, and to permit unsupervised chemoprophylaxis in all other individuals who might qualify.

At present isoniazid is the only drug for which controlled studies have been carried out to establish efficacy. Experimental data, however, indicate that the combination of rifampicin and pyrazinamide given intermittently for a period as short as 3 months may provide adequate chemoprophylaxis[9]. Should this be confirmed in clinical studies, it will obviously be of considerable importance for the prevention of tuberculous disease.

Drugs Used in Chemotherapy

The key drugs used in modern chemotherapy are isoniazid, rifampicin and pyrazinamide. When there is a high incidence of primary isoniazid resistance in an area, ethambutol will often be added to the regimen to help prevent the development of further resistance.

Other drugs which may be called upon in the presence of multi-drug resistance or drug toxicity include the aminoglycosides, streptomycin, amikacin and kanamycin, PAS and thiacetazone, quinalones such as ciprofloxacin, ofloxacin or sparfloxacin and ethionamide, prothionamide, cycloserine or capreomycin. Some of these drugs have a relatively high incidence of side effects and in most instances their place in the anti-tuberculosis regimen and their influence on the duration of therapy required is unclear. Any deviation from the standard regimen of isoniazid, rifampicin and pyrazinamide will, therefore, at present require an extension of the period of treatment from 6 months to 9 or even 18 months.

Isoniazid

Isoniazid has an excellent pharmacokinetic profile, and achieves more than adequate concentrations throughout the body, including the cerebrospinal fluid[20]. Genetically determined acetylation is the chief means of its excretion from the body and individuals can be typed as slow or fast acetylators, but this is not thought to have any significant effect on therapeutic efficacy[21].

Despite its proven efficacy in chemoprophylaxis isoniazid's main role is considered to be the rapid reduction in the mass of metabolically active organisms[2].

Besides hepatotoxicity and cutaneous hypersensitivity, isoniazid may also be responsible for peripheral neuropathy and more rarely for convulsions, psychoses, hemolytic or aplastic anemia and lupoid reactions[22].

Dosage: 5–10 mg/kg, to a maximum of 300 mg given in a single daily dose; or in intermittent therapy 15–20 mg/kg to a maximum of 900 mg.

Rifampicin

Rifampicin is a key drug in short-course chemotherapy and is particularly valued for its capacity to sterilize lesions. It is well tolerated in children and levels in excess of the minimal inhibitory concentration are achieved in the serum and most tissues when the drug is given in a single dose before breakfast.

Adverse effects are unusual in children but higher doses, especially when used in combination with isoniazid, have been associated with hepatitis. When used intermittently the so-called "flu syndrome" may occur and also rarely hemolytic anemia, thrombocytopenia, renal failure or dyspnea.

Dosage: 10 mg/kg, to a maximum of 600 mg in a single daily dose; 15–20 mg/kg in intermittent therapy, to a maximum of 600 mg.

Pyrazinamide

Following its development in 1949, pyrazinamide was initially used at a dosage of 50 mg/kg and was considered to be too hepatotoxic for routine use. It

is now used at a dose of approximately 35 mg/kg and is associated with very little toxicity in children. It has an important function in the sterilization of tuberculous lesions, due to its concentration in the acid intracellular environment of the macrophage.

Dosage: 30–35 mg/kg, in a single daily dose; 50 mg/kg in intermittent therapy, to a maximum of 2 g.

Ethambutol

This semi-synthetic drug bears no relationship to any of the other anti-tuberculosis drugs and no cross-resistance has been observed. It is not considered as a "first line" drug, but has a role in the prevention of drug resistance when given with other drugs. In areas with a high incidence of drug resistance it may also be included in routine regimens.

Although well tolerated it is associated with the development of retrobulbar neuritis, which occurs most frequently when ethambutol is used at higher doses over a long period of time. Although reversible and relatively infrequent it is not easy to evaluate children for this complication, so that ethambutol is not a drug of first choice in young children.

Dosage: 25 mg/kg for 2 months and then 15 mg for 4 months to a maximum of 150 mg; and 30–45 mg/kg in intermittent therapy.

Streptomycin

The aminoglycoside streptomycin acts mainly on metabolically active extracellular organisms, but contributes relatively little to the sterilization of lesions. It must be given by injection, which constitutes a considerable disadvantage in countries where HIV infection and AIDS are present. It remains a valuable drug which can be used in cases of drug resistance or toxicity to the other anti-tuberculosis drugs.

Drugs: 15–20 mg/kg in a single daily intramuscular injection to a maximum of 1 g.

Hepatotoxicity

Isoniazid, rifampicin and pyrazinamide may be responsible, individually or together for hepatotoxicity. A rise in liver enzyme levels (AST and ALT) to × 5 normal values is not uncommon following the start of therapy[23] and is presumed to be the result of enzyme induction. The occurrence of jaundice should, however, be viewed seriously and all therapy stopped immediately until the cause of the jaundice is clarified and the liver function tests have returned to normal. If considered necessary treatment may be continued in the interim with a combination of streptomycin and ethambutol which is unlikely to cause hepatotoxicity. Viral hepatitis is now considered to play an important predisposing role in many cases of hepatotoxicity and isoniazid, rifampicin and pyrazinamide can frequently be reintroduced without any complications[24].

Generalized and Cutaneous Hypersensitivity

Generalized and cutaneous hypersensitivity reactions can occur with any of the anti-tuberculosis drugs, but are fortunately rare in children. They may present with fever and be accompanied by a maculopapular or urticarial skin rash, lymphadenopathy and hepatosplenomegaly. In general, all treatment should stop and expert opinion sought in the management of these cases. Daily challenge doses of the relevant drugs may be required. Thiacetazone has caused severe cutaneous reactions when used to treat tuberculosis associated with HIV infection and AIDS. In those countries with a high incidence of HIV infection and AIDS thiacetazone should no longer be used for the treatment of tuberculosis.

Alternative Schedules and Regimes

In many countries daily supervised therapy is not feasible. Under these circumstances, intermittent therapy either twice weekly or three times weekly is used to facilitate supervision and to ease the task of clinic personnel. Under other circumstances, financial constraints may necessitate the use of alternative regimens and the omission of rifampicin. Any regimen that does not include rifampicin will have to be given for a period of at least 9 months or possibly longer, depending upon the precise combination of drugs used.

Experience in adults indicates that tuberculosis in HIV-infected individuals or those with AIDS can be treated for the same length of time as in non-infected individuals.

Extrapulmonary Tuberculosis

Controlled trials in most forms of extrapulmonary tuberculosis have confirmed that the same regimens used to treat pulmonary tuberculosis can be used for extrapulmonary tuberculosis. In the case of tuberculous meningitis anecdotal evidence suggests that therapy for 6 months will also suffice[25,26] but no published control trial has confirmed this. Also in tuberculous meningitis it is customary to use higher dosages of drugs to ensure sufficiently high concentrations are reached and maintained in the cerebrospinal fluid. Isoniazid 20 mg/kg, rifampicin 20 mg/kg and pyrazinamide 35 mg/kg are used, often augmented by ethionamide 20 mg/kg particularly in the presence of possible drug resistance. The necessity of the higher dosages in children is debatable, but the drugs are usually well tolerated in childhood.

Corticosteroids

In certain forms of tuberculosis such as pericarditis and pericardial effusion, corticosteroids have been shown in adults to have undoubted advantages[27]. Other situations in which the suppression of the inflammatory response may be advantageous include tuberculous meningitis, pleural effusion and enlarged mediastinal lymph nodes causing respiratory embarrassment[28]. Corticosteroids should never be used without the cover of effective anti-tuberculosis drugs. Depending upon the severity of the condition the dose of prednisone recommended is from 1 to 3 mg/kg and the dose should be increased by half should rifampicin be used. Corticosteroids should be continued for 1–2 months and then gradually withdrawn.

Drug Resistance

Despite earlier indications that drug-resistant mycobacteria might be less virulent, there is no doubt that such organisms can give rise to severe tuberculous disease. Failure to supervise chemotherapy has led to a dramatic rise in the incidence of drug-resistant tuberculosis throughout the world. Coupled to the association between HIV infection, AIDS and tuberculosis this has led to fears that tuberculosis could become unmanageable within the foreseeable future.

Primary or initial resistance occurs when the person is infected by drug-resistant organisms; while acquired or secondary resistance develops when a single drug is used, when two drugs are used and the infecting organisms are already resistant to one drug, or when a patient fails to take treatment as prescribed.

The key to the prevention of resistance lies in the supervision of therapy and the use of combination tablets making self-initiated monotherapy impossible.

In children drug-resistant tuberculosis will usually be primary resistance and should be suspected when the child comes from a country, neighbourhood or family with known drug resistance problems. In the presence of severe disease in such children it is prudent to add a fourth drug to the standard regimens (ethambutol or ethionamide) or to substitute an entirely new regimen depending upon the expected drug resistance patterns.

References

1. Smith MHD (1982). What about short course and intermittent chemotherapy for tuberculosis in children? Pediatr Infect Dis 1: 298–303
2. Mitchison DA (1985). The action of antituberculosis drugs in short course chemotherapy. Tubercle 66: 219–225
3. Mitchison DA, Dickinson JM (1978). Bactericidal mechanisms in short course chemotherapy. Bull IUATLD 53: 254–259
4. Sirgel FA, Botha FJH, Parkin DP, Van de Wal BW, Donald PR, Clark PK, Mitchison DA (1993). The early bactericidal activity of rifabutin in patients with pulmonary tuberculosis measured by sputum viable counts: a new method of drug assessment. J Antimicro Chemoth 32: 867–875
5. Grange JM (1990). Drug resistance and tuberculosis elimination. Bull IUAT 65: 57–59
6. Starke J (1990). Multidrug therapy for tuberculosis in children. Pediatr Infect Dis J 9: 785–793
7. Biddulph J, Kokaha V, Sharma S (1988). Short course chemotherapy in childhood tuberculosis. J Trop Ped 34: 20–23
8. Kumar L, Dhand R, Singhi PD, Rao KLN, Katariy S (1990). A randomized trial of fully intermittent vs daily followed by intermittent short course chemotherapy for childhood tuberculosis. Pediatr Infect Dis J 9: 802–806
9. Lecoeur HF, Truffot-Pernot C, Grosset JH (1989). Experimental short course preventative therapy of tuberculosis with rifampin and pyrazinamide. Am Rev Respir Dis 140: 1189–1193
10. Hong Kong Chest Service, Tuberculosis Research Centre, Madras, British MRC (1989). A controlled trial of 3-month, 4-month and 6-month regimens of chemotherapy for sputum-smear-negative pulmonary tuberculosis. Am Rev. Respir Dis 139: 871–876
11. Dutt AK, Moers D, Stead WW (1989). Smear- and culture-negative pulmonary tuberculosis: Four months short-course chemotherapy. Am Rev Respir Dis 139: 867–870
12. World Health Organization (1993). Treatment of tuberculosis. Guidelines for national programmes. Geneva: WHO
13. Chaulet P (1990/1991). Compliance with chemotherapy for tuberculosis. Responsibilities of the Health Ministry and of physicians. Bull IUAT Lung Dis 66 (Supplement): 33–35
14. Grzybowski S (1991). Tuberculosis in the third world. Thorax 46: 689–691
15. Brudney K, Dobkin J (1991). Resurgent tuberculosis in New York city. Human immunodeficiency virus, homelessness and the decline of tuberculosis control programmes. Am Rev Respir Dis 144: 745–749
16. Farer LS (1982). Chemoprophylaxis. Am Rev. Respir Dis 125: 102–107
17. Lincoln EM (1950). Course and prognosis of tuberculosis in children. Am J Med 9: 623–632
18. Rouillon A, Perdrizet S, Parrot R (1976). Transmission of tubercle bacilli: the effects of chemotherapy. Tubercle 57: 257–299
19. Wallgren A (1948). The time-table of tuberculosis. Tubercle 29: 245–251
20. Donald PR, Gent WL, Seifart HI, Lamprecht JH, Parkin DP (1992). Cerebrospinal fluid isoniazid concentrations in children with tuberculous meningitis: the influence of dosage and acetylation status. Pediatrics 89: 247–250
21. Ellard GA (1984). The potential clinical significance of the isoniazid anetylator phenotype in the treatment of pulmonary tuberculosis. Tubercle 65: 211–250
22. Girling DJ (1982). Adverse effects of antituberculosis drugs. Drugs 23: 56–74
23. Donald PR, Schoeman JF, O'Kennedy A (1987). Hepatic toxicity during chemotherapy for severe tuberculous meningitis. Am J Dis Child 141: 741–743
24. Kumar A, Misra PK, Mehotra R et al (1991). Hepatotoxicity of rifampicin and isoniazid. Am Rev Respir Dis 143: 1350–1352
25. Lorber J (1960). Treatment of tuberculous meningitis. Lancet 1: 1309–1312
26. Kending EL, Burch CD (1960). Short-term antimicrobial therapy of tuberculous meningitis. Am Rev Respir Dis 82: 672–681
27. Strang JIG, Kakaza HHS, Gibson DG et al (1982). Controlled trial of prednisone as adjuvant in treatment of tuberculous constrictive pericarditis in Transkei. Lancet 2: 1418–1422
28. Alzeer AH, Fritz JM (1993). Corticosteroids and tuberculosis: risks and use as adjunct therapy. Tubercle Lung Dis 74: 6–11

Subject Index